Osteopathy for Children

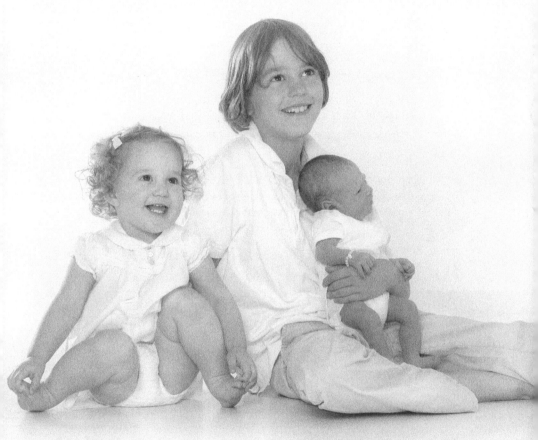

Holistic and Natural Treatments for the Developing Infant, Toddler & Growing Child

LeTrinh Hoang, D.O.

Hatherleigh Press is committed to preserving and protecting the natural resources of the earth. Environmentally responsible and sustainable practices are embraced within the company's mission statement.

Visit us at www.hatherleighpress.com and register online for free offers, discounts, special events, and more.

Library of Congress Cataloging-in-Publication Data is available.

ISBN: 978-1-57826-615-9

BOOK DESIGN BY CAROLYN KASPER

CONTENTS

PART III:
MEDICAL PROBLEMS WITH STRUCTURAL CAUSES 89

PART IV:
HOW TO HELP OR FIND HELP FOR YOUR CHILD 149

INTRODUCTION

W HILE I was in the clinical clerkship phase of my osteopathic schooling, I was fairly certain that I would be pursuing a pediatric residency. I had even picked one out: the M.D. program at Loma Linda University Children's Hospital was very osteopathy friendly. But because the training program was intense, and I had no D.O. (Doctor of Osteopathy) mentors, I ended up dedicating very little time to truly understanding the meaning and power of what traditional, hands-on treatment of the physical body can accomplish.

It was only after I had worked for other pediatricians, and later when I established my own office, that I began to see, not just the cracks, but gaping holes in how we treat children. It was then that I returned to the study of traditional osteopathy. I had an urgent care contract with a local HMO, through which I saw lots of children, many of whom would come back frequently for the same types of infections. We in turn would give them the same medicines over and over again, but, we never really resolved the cause of their chronic, recurrent problems.

As I was relearning osteopathy, I would have patients come in and complain of ailments like ear infections. While I thought that I should try to help them *my way* with osteopathy, I would give antibiotics for the ear infection, just in case. I did not think that I would hear back from the patient or find out what happened as a result: it would only be a year or so later that I would get feedback, with parents telling me, "You did that one thing and our child didn't need to have ear tubes put in." Then more years would pass and then more people would come in saying, "My friend said you did this, that you cured them of this..."

I am still amazed by what patients and parents tell me. Although it seems hard to believe, done just right, results *are* instantaneous.

The purpose of this book is twofold: to guide parents and adult patients who continue to search for answers, and to inspire a new generation of physicians to see and do the impossible.

OVERVIEW: THE LOST ART

I N T H E United States, there are 144 allopathic schools and 30 osteopathic schools that educate doctors in the practice of medicine.
Various government data and statistics report that the total number of
physicians attending to patients amounts roughly to 770,000 clinicians.
Of this number, osteopathic physicians (D.O.) number about 75,000,
roughly 9.7 percent of the total number of physicians in practice. Of
those 75,000 D.O. physicians in the United States, only about 5 percent
practice osteopathic medicine the way it was originally intended by the
founder of the profession, Andrew Taylor Still, M.D.

Dr. Still opened the first osteopathic school in 1892 with the intent
of teaching medicine in a new way, completely different from his allopathic training. In his time, medicine was still quite unorganized. He
criticized the disease-oriented approach. His philosophy was to find the
patient's *health,* because as he put it, "Anyone can find disease." In fact,
disease should be viewed as the endpoint of a long process of disorder,
strain, and injury. To recover the patient and return them to health, a
doctor must first reverse that process and undo the strain or injury. Dr.
Still's idea was revolutionary; it is the body's design and balance that is
responsible for our good health; disease results when the body's natural
balance is constrained by injuries, strains, and displacements.

As I understand it, the mechanically unrestricted body is balanced
and efficient, the result of which is good health and a reduced susceptibility to disease. Very few doctors understand this, and even less
practice it. Of the roughly 75,000 D.O. physicians in practice, only about
3,700 of us practice traditional osteopathy. It is for this reason that I call
traditional osteopathy a Lost Art, compounded by the fact that we do

not publicize our results, and there is very little written about how we actually treat our patients. In addition, many patients who refer a friend or family member to a traditional osteopathic practice set for them a very high expectation of miraculous change, one that we often cannot fulfill. Knowing what injury pattern a patient carries is never a certainty, and even they sometimes do not know for sure.

My mentor, Herb Miller, D.O., who was well known in our world and much sought after for teaching conferences, never left any writings. I believe that I will follow his path; I don't believe I will ever write a manual on how the art of osteopathy is done. However, I *do* believe that patients all over the world (who are still searching for answers), as well as students and even clinicians need to see a compendium of treatment effects and all the wondrous possibilities of this lost art.

Within these pages are a few of my patients before and after treatment photos. The lost art of traditional osteopathy, as practiced by an experienced physician, will result in instantaneous reduction in tissue tension and visible changes soon thereafter. Quite often, these changes themselves are instantaneous, as well. These changes continue throughout the course of a week as the body corrects itself and restores its natural balance. Each treatment augments the prior treatment, until the body is whole and healthy.

PART I

TRADITIONAL OSTEOPATHY

PART I: OVERVIEW

More often than not, traumatic injuries impart vectors and strains *on the whole body*. Partial resolution of vectors, regardless of the means used to treat them, is still partial. In other words, partial (and perhaps imprecise) reduction of traumatic vectors will still leave partially treated strains in place, which will need to be dealt with later. Suppose an adult is in a rear-end collision, which causes blunt facial trauma when the head hits the steering wheel, followed by whiplash when the back of the head hits the headrest. Any therapeutic technique which only addresses the face would therefore be inadequate. Furthermore, how would a limited technique address the traumatic vectors in the lower back, which can go on to cause back pain, spasms, and even a bulging disc? Traditional osteopathy, with its focus on the whole, as opposed to the tunnel vision that can result from local technique, is better suited to dealing with the systemic, global nature of traumatic injury. This is especially true for children, in whom partial treatment will only alter the injury pattern. As the untreated parts develop into an adult structure, their pain will return, worse than before. The contrast is clear—the advantage that osteopathy has over allopathy is one of *perspective*.

CHAPTER 1

History of
Traditional Osteopathy

NDREW TAYLOR Still was an army physician, living and practicing on the frontier—first in Kansas and later in Missouri. Upon
his return from the Civil War at the age of 36, three of his children
had already died of spinal meningitis in an epidemic. Two weeks later,
a fourth child died of pneumonia. The deaths of his children must have
presented a professional crisis, because Dr. Still began to study spiritu-
alism, magnetic healing, and bone setting. By the time he was 46 years
old, he was ready to present his ideas. He saw failings in the medicine
of his day. He saw that the treatments then, as now, addressed only the
symptoms of illness. He felt that if the *cause* of a person's ailment could
be found and addressed, then the effects would resolve themselves. He
reasoned that "the architecture of the God of Nature" in health meant
"perfection and harmony, not in one part, but in the whole."

Dr. Still and his research were publicly rejected. He continued to
develop and practice his brand of mechanical medicine, a system which
he termed osteopathy. In 1892, at the age of 64, Dr. Still saw the first
school of osteopathy open its doors to students.

For more reading on the history of Andrew Taylor Still, the remarkable founder of the osteopathic profession, I recommend Steven Paulus Osteopathy at http://osteopathichistory.com. Also see: *The Lengthening Shadow of Andrew Taylor Still* (by Arthur Grant Hildreth), *Autobiography of Andrew Taylor Still, Philosophy and Mechanical Principles of Osteopathy,* and *Osteopathy: Research and Practice.*

CHAPTER 2

Philosophy of Traditional Osteopathy

T HE PHILOSOPHICAL approach of an osteopathic treatment is unlike any other conventional or ancillary health approach. It stands alone in its focus on finding health and balance, as opposed to finding "disease." One of Dr. Still's most enduring admonitions was to "find the health"; he reasoned that anyone can "find disease." Osteopathy is the only medical philosophy that does not assert force or an expectation of what a body or patient should be; it does not attempt to change the patient to suit preexisting expectations. Because it is a mechanical philosophy, the problems that a patient presents are often viewed as the result of multiple accumulated mechanical disruptions and displacements over time. Because the body is functionally a unit, composed of the interworking of multiple systems, a local problem does not always have a local cause. The actual cause may be remote, dispersing tensions along and out toward the rest of the body. With a minor injury, the body adapts to the injury by spreading out the tensions and returns itself to the relative normal functions of walking and moving about. When a body acquires more injuries, its ability to distribute tensions remotely and balance itself becomes more difficult. When the body can no longer adapt, the patient feels pain. When pain is present, it affects the patient's functioning; the body can no longer accommodate the accumulated injuries and the patient has decompensated. Osteopathy is unique, because hands-on diagnosis and treatment are focused on removing or reducing the traumatic strain trapped in the muscle and tissue memory of the body. Removal of traumatic strains allows the body to balance tensions and return to its normal function prior to injury.

CHAPTER 3

Comparison to Conventional Allopathic Care

A s MOST patients come to see over time, there are many reasons why traditional osteopathy is considered so different and distinct from conventional, allopathic medicine. The primary difference between osteopathy and conventional medicine is that, in primary care, M.D.s use their hands purely for physical exams, as one element in their diagnostic procedure. By contrast, traditional D.O.s use their hands for both diagnosis and treatment.

Another difference is what can be called the "temporal association." In conventional medicine, when there is a problem, whether it is an injury to treat or a disease to diagnose, the patient is presented as such. In other words, conventional medicine looks at a patient presenting with symptoms as being the result of the patient's current condition; the problem is dealt with as being in the here-and-now.

With traditional osteopathy, we take the patient back to the time of the injury by—as my mentor used to say—"engaging" the tissue. Once the tissue is "engaged," we apply work to "disengage" it. Traumatized tissue lives and functions with (oftentimes in *spite* of) the memory of injury. Take, for example, a simple minor slip and fall injury onto the tailbone. The fall induces an upward compression force from the buttocks into the low back. The bones are jammed up, and the muscles deep in the pelvis that attach to these bones seize up and spasm. They spasm for two reasons: (1) because of the shock of the trauma; and (2) because the bones are jammed up together, the muscle ends are now *shortened*. The normal resting lengths of these muscles have actually been altered. Often, falls on the buttocks affect the psoas muscles. The psoas (pronounced SO-AZ) is a long muscle on both sides of our body that attaches from the last floating rib, runs deep in our waist behind the intestines, down through the pelvis and attaches to our thigh bone. It is the main muscle we use to lift our leg up, an action called hip flexion. We need hip flexion to walk up stairs, to get up from a seated position, to swing one leg up and forward as we walk. Because this muscle is shortened through involuntary contraction from the trauma, it is already "engaged." This is why after a fall, it is painful to walk and most people limp. The muscle cannot relax and lengthen, which is necessary to allow for another action of lifting or flexing the hip. To relieve the pain and allow for relaxation, osteopaths have to find that muscle and "disengage" it by further shortening the shortened muscle, and then lengthening it. If left alone, over time the tissue and muscle will remodel themselves after this new, artificially shortened length, as the body comes to accept it as "normal." When treating a fall on or around the buttocks and tailbone, I check to see if the psoas is contracted and painful. However old the injury, I treat the muscle, tissue, and bone as if it happened today.

Osteopaths are trained to apply enough work to address the issue, and nothing more—we strive to use only what the patient needs, and not more (otherwise, we would induce additional strain). The key is to match whatever tension it is that they and their tissue need at that time. Naturally, this is exceptionally high-precision work, requiring the osteopath to change and respond to the patient as they change and respond to the treatment. The interaction and the treatment are both highly dynamic. After the treatment, the osteopath has to balance the released tension. Once an injured tissue is freed up, because of the elastic nature of living tissue, it will "bounce" the other way into freedom, and then back again toward the old injury pattern of restriction. I call this the

Rubberbanding Effect. The tissue toggles back and forth between its recent pathological injured state and the prior memory of the "normal" it used to know. Balancing and rebalancing tissue tensions are important for the patient's sense of well-being following a treatment. This is the only field of medicine that seeks not to "do," but rather tries to "undo." A good osteopathic treatment does not invade and, although this can be difficult, should not even "assert."

Another example of how an M.D. and a D.O. differ in the understanding of disease is the herniated disc. If a patient with back pain has a herniated disc measuring 5 millimeters, most conventional M.D. and D.O. surgeons will start talking about surgery. They know the anatomy and the structure of the lumbar spine; they understand that this patient has endured some significant degree of trauma as to cause instability. The surgery will require cutting, plates and screws, and bone grafting or cleaning tissue debris in the area. The distinction here between the conventional and traditional D.O. approach is that the trauma from so many years ago, the one that got the patient to this point, is not typically addressed by conventional medicine. After surgery, the tissue area scars and tightens up. While it is actually stable, it remains stiff. The traumatic strain (the cause of the instability) from a years-old accident is still in place. Years after a back surgery, it isn't uncommon to see the discs above and below the area of the operation become weakened and start to herniate. The time it takes to affect adjacent segments depends on the degree of force; the harder and more violent the impact, the sooner that the other areas are affected. For lumbar discs, the patients who consult me report the return of their symptoms occurring between 7 and 10 years after a back surgery.

This temporal understanding, this appreciation of the timeline of tissue injury, is one of the secrets of traditional osteopathy. The key lies in understanding that, just because an injury occurred in the past doesn't mean that it *stays* in the past. In evaluating a patient, we take a medical history. An osteopath understands that today's complaints and problems have everything to do with how our bodies adapt to old injuries. Ultimately, in seeking to free the patient from needing medical assistance or pharmaceutical intervention, we address every significant past injury.

ALLOPATHIC VS. OSTEOPATHIC EDUCATION

As osteopaths, how and what we learn about the human body and its workings is also strikingly different from the typical M.D. curriculum. Generally, in medicine, academia, and any STEM (science, technology, engineering, and math) field, when looking at how to scientifically arrive at a conclusion, we need evidence. We need to prove the theory by designing controlled experiments and studies. For example, when seeking to understand how biological systems work or how physiology works, we study animal models and conduct experiments. This data helps us prove or disprove a theory. Just as importantly, the data needs to be reproducible, and drawn from a large enough statistical sample so that we can have confidence in the results.

For traditional osteopathic physicians, this is difficult to do. The problems or diseases that osteopaths examine are dependent on each individual's history of prior traumas. It would be difficult, if not impossible, to create a sample size large enough and homogenous enough to satisfy scientific rigor. And even if such a sample group were available, the study results would be difficult to duplicate and prove, because techniques and treatment styles vary from physician to physician. Take car accidents, for example. Two people rear-ended at a stop sign in different accidents *will* most likely have whiplash from front to back, and or else back to front. But the *medical problems* of soft tissue injury several weeks later will not be the same. If one person has had a prior neck injury, they will suffer far more from the same force of whiplash, as compared to a person with no prior neck trauma. Animal models could never work, because no animal model can match the postural mechanics and gravitational loads of weight bearing of two-legged human beings. (Fortunately, large medical centers and affiliated teaching institutions, both allopathic and osteopathic, *are* attempting to do this research, and continue to call for more studies.) Granted, these are mostly my professional opinions, but they are based on clinical experience and are commonly shared by my colleagues in private practice.

Most of our education comes about through hands-on experience, learning directly from our patients. What does a strain feel like? What does a vector feel like? A vector is a force with direction. Injured tissue has a specific *feel*. When we apply pressure through our fingers to counter and reduce an old trauma, the tissue transforms underneath our hands. We can *sense* the force of the initial injury and which way it went, which is *implied* by the instantaneous change in the tissue. The tissue gets softer and the patient often reports it feeling "lighter." What changes happen to tissues as we reduce a vector? How does this affect the way the tissue feels, and how does this particular body adapt? I often tell my patients that the physical laws governing the universe apply to our bodies as well. We are not so special that we can defy them; the mystery is rather how our biological systems *adapt* to these physical laws. One of the secrets of traditional osteopathy is figuring out and unlocking those adaptations after the body begins to decompensate.

THE PATIENT'S PERCEPTION

Even my regular patients have difficulty explaining the concepts that I teach them. When they try to explain to their family and friends, they usually end up resorting to statements like, "I don't know what she does, but it works." Another patient will say, "She does this, this, and this (making patting motions with their open palms) and you're all better!" When one patient told me she had actually said this to a friend she wanted to refer, I cringed internally. I asked her to not explain osteopathy in such a mystical way; in fact, I would rather that she does not explain it at all. Osteopathy is not mysticism. In the past, some patients have described my work on them as "voodoo," "magic," "miraculous," even "God's work." The reason that they cannot comprehend osteopathy as a scientific art is due to its subtlety. When I was first starting out, in my first 7 years of relearning osteopathy, I was sweating bullets moving arms and legs, positioning and repositioning myself and the patient. All the gross mechanical work I did took twice as long and achieved only half as much as what I can accomplish today. The secret is precision. When the work is precise, there is less work to be done and less force needed to do it. This precision comes from a refined ability to put concepts into practice.

FEELING AND SENSING

From the first day of osteopathic school, we are taught about *palpation,* or the act of finding specific tissue areas with our hands. All medical schools teach their students how to perform a physical exam and feel for pathological changes in the body. For example, we are taught to look and feel for lumps in the breasts, cysts underneath the skin, or stool lodged in the constipated colon. But the osteopathic palpatory experience goes further than just finding lumps and bumps where they don't belong. We are taught to feel for spasms in the muscles, local tensions in ligaments and tendons, and even tissue tensions far away from the injury site. We are taught to think along the lines of: "Something has happened to this patient's body, and it is now altered." In the physical exam, we try to feel for what is wrong. For new patients, I often find a spastic muscle and press on it with my fingertip. I would identify it and say, "There it is." An acute spasm has a fast contraction rate. A chronic or old spasm has a boggy tissue feel and a slower contraction rate. I use my hands, opening and closing my fingers to demonstrate the rate. The timing of my hands is matched to the patient's contraction rate so they know that I do actually know what they are feeling.

As we continue to more advanced coursework (usually after the seventh year), we have the option to continue learning about sensory experience as it relates to the treatment of patients. We learn to sense changes in the tissue. We put our hands on the tissue and observe what it does. Its repetitive action implies a traumatic vector. A vector is simply a force with a direction. If a body part feels like it is moving in one direction, it has either done it multiple times in the past (e.g., a repetitive stress injury) or, if it *was* only done once, it was done with extreme *force* (e.g., a high velocity deceleration injury). Either way, the tissue is caught and stuck in that movement memory. I like to say that it "lives" in the memory of the injury. It still "thinks" that it is moving left or right, or that the leg is still kicking, and so on. I recall asking one of my patients, "Why does it seem like your left leg wants to kick?" He responded that the left leg was his kicking leg when he studied karate for 3 years. Another patient was a former European kickboxing champion. At age 45, he had been diagnosed by a neurologist as having "restless leg syndrome." I told him that the problem with his leg was not that it is "restless," but rather that it was too effectively trained to kick; it thinks that it has still been kicking for the last 20 years, despite my patient having been retired all that time. In high precision treatment, we sense what a tissue does, in order to determine the force at work. Once we reduce a vector and feel the tissue change, we also sense that the force dissipates, transforms, or "releases." In effect, we are taught to sense *energetic shifts* as a tissue's traumatic vector is reduced.

THE "ENERGY" PHILOSOPHY OF TRADITIONAL OSTEOPATHY

This "energy" aspect of traditional osteopathy is very esoteric, and still hidden to most osteopathic physicians, who practice only conventional medicine. Even within our professional organizations and associations, the way in which this energy concept is taught—and even if it should be taught at all—remains a controversial subject. Some of my colleagues refuse to acknowledge it at all. Even my mentor Dr. Miller chose not to recognize or teach anything but anatomical and mechanical concepts. I only found this secret path of traditional osteopathy in much the same way most of my patients find me—not through advertisement, but through word of mouth. It has taken me 7 years to acknowledge that there is an energy component to why my patients improve. For the longest time, I refused to even mention the "E" word in explaining to my patients how I am able to feel the changes in their body *without* putting my hands on their body, and further discussion on this esoteric energy aspect of traditional osteopathy deserves its own book. Needless to say, it forms a core part of my treatment approach, and I consider it a valuable tool in my practice.

ADVANCED COURSE WORK

In our advanced course work (well beyond the basic mechanics of structure) we invariably come to the ultimate questions of how we arrive at the human adult structure. The patient before us has a whole history of acquired traumas, going all the way back to their childhood. Even before infancy, there may be traumatic forces at play, in our earliest formation. The question of how to achieve results for patients can take us back that far. Ultimately, I believe that the work I do is heavily invested in embryology, the study of how the human body forms, and how living biological systems adapt to traumatic forces while still obeying physical laws. How we come to be at any moment in time and how everything that has happened to our physical body is involved and invested in everything that will happen, is the crux of osteopathy. When a body has advanced past the point of full-on "disease," it takes much longer and requires more cumulative work to return it to balance so that it may make its own recovery.

We are taught to thank our patients for allowing us to learn from them, and as I was relearning osteopathy, I came to realize that this teaching is correct, and comes from physicians who have experienced a lifetime of learning, thanks to the cooperation of their patients. For many years at the start of osteopathy's history, traditional osteopaths had to endure rejection, ridicule, and prejudicial treatment from their allopathic colleagues, and even from those within the profession itself. Thankfully, the tide is slowly starting to change; I have come to understand that my own prior narrow-mindedness was impeding my development, both personally and professionally. These teachings, passed down through generations of osteopaths, deserve to be preserved and continued—hence, this book.

HUGGING AND HUMILITY

When I first transitioned from my basic course work to more advanced osteopathy studies, I observed a huge social difference in physician to patient interaction, as well as collegial interaction. It was quite shocking; I found myself often thinking, with incredulity, "What is with all the hugging?" It seemed to me to be an affront to my sensibilities; in my conventional medical training, I was conditioned to create a wall of separation between people in day-to-day interactions.

After 15 years of osteopathic work, that initial impression has been flipped. Whereas the fast-paced world of conventional medicine rarely allows time for such niceties, the work we do requires time and patience. And patients appreciate the time we spend with them—the results are the reward. However, having gone through this myself, seeing both worlds through the lens of human interaction, I do not believe those worlds can merge. They are separate, and must remain separate; it is up to the patients to make a choice as to which professional atmosphere they prefer.

In interactions with teachers, mentors and experienced physicians, I have observed the greatest possible humility in the most skilled, talented, and gifted among us. I have come to understand that this humility comes with a hard-earned wisdom and a wealth of secret knowledge. It has been my experience that the wisest and most skilled among us eventually stop talking; they let others confirm their skills and convince the skeptics. Above all, they leave very little behind. My personal sentiment is that there should be more of us quietly doing this great work. Anyone who seeks answers, who seeks us out for our skills and services, *will* find us. I have come to agree with my teachers in that we should just do our work, while we teach others the ideas, concepts, and philosophy. We do not teach "how-to" techniques; there should never be any manuals published with instructions for where to put which fingers, and how to do this or that. These would simply be recipe books. Understanding the broader concepts of the mechanical human body and how injuries can throw it out of balance allows the physician to come up with his or her own "techniques," which are almost universally more effective than a cookie-cutter, one-size-fits-all version of osteopathy.

LEARNING THE BASICS

With basic course work, we learn the oldest and most fundamental "techniques" of our profession. As we advance and develop our own style, we share our own, newly-developed techniques with each other. For example: my mentor, Dr. Herb Miller, was well known for having an amazing maneuver for resetting the sacrum perfectly between the ilia (the two hip bones). He was very well respected in our field, and in high demand for teaching courses. His movements were so easy, fluid, and graceful that one would be forgiven for thinking that he didn't do very much. The secret was his precision. The patient would get up after receiving treatment, and their gait would be completely changed. His technique was effective for back spasms, and even patients with herniated discs and jammed and stuck sacroiliac joints. I had a conversation with him about his maneuver and the reasons why it was so powerful and effective. I called it the Herb Miller Technique, and told him how I would use it for my husband, modify it for use on myself, and even present a simplified version as an exercise for my patients.

Of course, Dr. Miller never identified the things he did as being his "technique"; he did not offer seminars in how to imitate his movements. Rather, it was through observing his treatment, watching where he palpated the patient's anatomic landmarks, and the sequence in which he did it, that I was able to incorporate it into my repertoire. As I said, osteopathy is primarily an experiential brand of medicine, both in terms of the physician and their patients. So, when we share "techniques" and discuss methodology, it isn't meant to represent "absolute gold standards," something that is passed on. These discussions span questions of what, why, and where; the one question that should never be asked is, "How?" While attempting to answer that question may well lead to a demonstration, which would be to the benefit of those observing, it would likely result in a step-by-step explication, accompanied by furious note-taking, all of which could lead to the unwarranted and unwanted "recipe book" of osteopathy.

When we compare the allopathic world to the osteopathic world, the differences are almost too vast to contemplate. The two fields are distinct and separate, and must remain so. For osteopaths, the need for scientific proof of efficacy is not a major drive, because the philosophy is rooted in the basic science of human anatomy and functional, mechanical principles. Our professional and economic survival is purely results driven. After gaining experience, results and wisdom, we no longer seek proof, and we leave no proof. This is why the mystery of traditional osteopathy remains hidden.

CHAPTER 4

Comparison to Other Manual Therapies

T HE PURPOSE of this section is to inform patients about other medical modalities are available, and to provide a pediatrician and traditional osteopathic physician's perspective on these alternative methods of care. It is *not* the goal of this chapter to either endorse or oppose these other types of therapies. The benefit of this insight is that, with a pediatrician's eye toward how a young child's body should develop, parents can more readily assess and anticipate normal development. If development does not occur as expected, I usually recommend a conservative observation period. After all, it does no harm to observe how a child's musculoskeletal system unfolds. The adult body ultimately forms and eventually walks, and can still be deduced, reduced, and treated (although the older the cause, the more visits it will take to see results).

Insurance companies often confuse and confound these differing approaches by lumping them together under the banner of manual therapy approaches. However, osteopathy is not a manual therapy—it isn't even the "master of all manual therapies." No other therapeutic approach will result in instantaneous changes of the bony facial structures and soft tissues, or reduction of muscular and postural tensions. It is a system of medicine that can sustain, and is sustained *by,* an understanding of the human body and how disease comes about.

PHYSICAL THERAPY

Physical therapy as an established profession has a long history. It got its start in the late 1800s, when programs were first developed to teach physical therapy education—among them the Sargent School, started by Dudley Allen Sargeant, M.D. The school had an affiliation with Harvard University, and sought to teach students physical examination involving measurements that now would be called vital signs, personal history, and health history. After this history was gathered and the patient's current status verified, specific exercises would then be prescribed.

Schools continued to spring up around the country, one after another. One school of physical education, the Boston Normal School of Gymnastics, was started by two women, Mary Hemenway and Amy Homans. Graduates of this school started another school, the Boston School of Physical Education. The programs and schools continued to expand, both in number and in scope, as course work continued to increase. It was clear that there was a need and demand for recovering the physical body with exercise and movement.

Physical therapy (and occupational therapy) as a profession really began to receive recognition after America became involved in World War I. Those wounded in the war needed to be quickly triaged for rehabilitation in order to return them to the battlefield as soon as possible. Those who could not return were transferred back to the United States, where they received physical therapy from graduates of the aforementioned schools and programs. At that time, physical therapy primarily consisted of exercise, massage, hydrotherapy, and electrotherapy. The goal was to physically restore as much function as possible to the injured body.

For more information on the history of physical therapy, the best resource is The American Physical Therapy Association. *Healing the Generations: A History of Physical Therapy and the American Physical Therapy Association* by Wendy B. Murphy, which was commissioned by the APTA itself, is a well-researched and wonderful read for anyone interested in manual therapy.

Today, according to the Bureau of Labor Statistics there are over 200,000 physical therapists in active practice (this estimate does not include practitioners who are self-employed).[1] Within the physical therapy profession, there is also an increase in specialization, with several schools in the United States offering doctorate training. As in the past, and conventionally today, the profession uses multiple modalities to help the patient return to normal functioning. These modalities include the well-established use of exercises for strength and balance, manual therapies (including massage), and hydrotherapy (which includes whirlpool and aquatic therapy). Hot and cold therapy and traction are also established mainstay treatments. Ultrasound therapy, light therapy, transcutaneous electrical nerve stimulation (TENS), and iontophoresis (the local delivery of medication using an electrical charge) are newer modalities, just now coming into practice.

In clinical practice, traditional osteopaths usually see patients after they have been through physical therapy. On occasion, after reducing the traumatic strains from an injury, I will refer a patient to physical therapy if I feel that the patient needs more work on strength and balance. Other patients, on recommendation from their M.D., choose to pursue physical therapy and osteopathy simultaneously. These are usually well-established patients who understand what they are getting from each professional.

The traditional osteopathic physician diagnoses and treats with use of the hands, without the use of any diagnostic or therapeutic devices. The philosophy is the modality—as one of our most famous teachers

William Garner Sutherland would say, "Good old-fashioned ten-finger osteopathy" is all we need.

Insurance companies, for labeling purposes, consider osteopathic treatments as a "physical therapy." However, for insurance purposes, for legal reasons, and because of differences in training, physical therapists cannot say that they are rendering osteopathic treatments. Because of the differences apparent in both philosophy and treatment approach, I suspect even physical therapists would agree that traditional osteopathy should not be categorized as a subset of physical therapy; rather, osteopathy should be seen as a medical philosophy.

CHIROPRACTIC

The chiropractic profession was started by a magnetic healer named D. D. Palmer in 1895. Since he opened the Palmer School of Chiropractic in 1897, the profession has grown to include an estimated 65,000 chiropractors in practice today and 16 chiropractic colleges in the United States.[2]

The main philosophical treatment focus of chiropractic is the correction of a subluxation. A subluxation is a misalignment of a bony vertebral spinal segment, usually corrected through chiropractic adjustments.[3] Chiropractors frequently use plain film x-rays or biomechanical analysis to diagnose injuries, which may include range of motion measurements as well as functional and physical performance evaluations. Treatment modalities primarily include adjustment techniques. Other physical treatment modalities include heat, ice, and electrotherapies such as ultrasound, interferential (current) therapy, and TENS (transcutaneous electrical nerve stimulation, a form of electrotherapy). Chiropractors also prescribe exercises and diet and lifestyle counseling.[4] According to the American Chiropractic Association, other accepted treatment modalities are massage, light therapy with lasers, acupuncture, and craniosacral therapy.[5]

Manual therapies and their treatment modalities are starting to cross over. Physical therapy is considered the first line conventional approach to muscular problems and rehabilitation, and is usually the first referral from a conventional allopathic physician. Patients who choose chiropractic, by contrast, usually go directly, without consulting an allopathic physician. Other than the spinal adjustment, chiropractic has some of the same modalities as physical therapy.

Also the training of D.O.s and D.C.s is significantly different. Most of our training is medical, and comparable to D.C.s. Most of our residency programs are hospital based where both M.D.s and D.O.s. work side by side. Rarely do D.O.s come in contact with D.C.s at the residency level, or in private practice for that matter.

As a conventionally trained general pediatrician, I do not agree with high velocity adjustments of the cervical spine for infants and children. I do not even agree with gentle craniosacral therapy for infants and children. Nor do I agree with chiropractic preventative wellness adjustments or preventative wellness craniosacral therapy. Philosophically, the idea of preventative wellness adjustments goes against the core osteopathic concept that the mechanically balanced body is "perfection and harmony." If an infant or child is doing well clinically, and is without any problems, he or she is healthy and does not require treatments. The presumption that a chiropractor can detect a problem *before* it becomes a problem, or that they can determine when an imbalance is soon to take place, is highly troublesome for me. It implies that the patient cannot tell when they will have a problem, as well as implying a lifetime of dependence on adjustments, which is antithetical to the traditional osteopathic approach of undoing what has been done, so that the mechanical body is free and unrestricted to balance and recover its health on its own.

I generally advise waiting for problems to occur so that, whatever therapy the parent has chosen for their child, they can directly observe the results. When a parent has chosen a treatment approach, my role is to function as a general pediatrician offering primary care services. For example, if a parent chooses to go to a pediatric neurologist and is satisfied with the two prescription medications for her teen daughter with migraine, my role is supportive. If the migraines continue and worsen,

I do not try to manage the medication; instead, I refer them back to their specialist. The same is true in the case of chiropractic: if a parent has already chosen structural work for their child, whether physical therapy, chiropractic, or craniosacral therapy, I do not offer my services for traditional osteopathy. My role is supportive as a general pediatrician. It is my position that the philosophy of chiropractic is largely incompatible with the philosophy of traditional osteopathy.

CRANIOSACRAL THERAPY

Craniosacral therapy, or CST, is a registered trademark of the Upledger Institute, a company founded by John Upledger, D.O. He was an osteopathic physician and a professor of biomechanics who taught at the College of Osteopathic Medicine at the State University of Michigan. He started his Upledger Institute to teach his philosophical anatomic approach of the craniosacral system. Oftentimes, CST-certified practitioners are physical therapists, licensed massage therapists, chiropractors, PhDs, and licensed acupuncturists. Very rarely do I see medical physicians teaching or practicing craniosacral therapy. CST is a gentle, hands-on method of evaluating and enhancing the functioning of a physiological body system called the craniosacral system comprised of the membranes and cerebrospinal fluid that surround and protect the brain and spinal cord.[6]

Many patients who have heard of craniosacral therapy, and who know that it was started by an osteopathic physician, ask me how much CST I use in my treatments. My response is: none. My explanation is that the education and training between a traditional osteopath and a CST practitioner are different, although some parents need to see this for themselves. I often advise parents that, before taking their children for craniosacral therapy, they should perhaps schedule a visit for themselves.

From a pediatrician's perspective, I believe that infants and children should be approached more conservatively. What may work gently and well for adults may not for infants and children, as their bodies are still developing. Infants and children are not easier to treat because they are softer—they are *more* difficult because they are as yet unformed. I generally do not offer traditional osteopathy services to patients who have had craniosacral therapy—it just creates more work. As gentle as it is, the original infant strain pattern has been altered. Now that someone else has worked on it, it requires more work to try and get back to the injury's original pattern. It is my experience that pediatric patients who have had CST do not respond instantaneously to my style of traditional osteopathy, which is what leads me to conclude that the original strain pattern is now altered.

NEUROMUSCULAR THERAPY

Neuromuscular therapy (NMT) is a form of manual therapy focusing on soft tissue which originated in Europe in the 1930s and 1940s. Leon Chaitow, D.O., nephew of one of the original founders of neuromuscular therapy (Boris Chaitow, DO), developed these techniques further while in England, and by the 1990s NMT was being taught as an elective model at the University of Westminster in London. In the United States, courses taught on neuromuscular therapy are primarily open to licensed massage therapists. The main focus is the treatment of myofascial trigger points, acute injuries, and chronic pain.[7] While I have not yet encountered patients who have undergone NMT in my practice, this philosophy is included here because manual therapies as a whole tend to use massage as a treatment technique.

MASSAGE THERAPY

According to the Bureau of Labor Statistics, as of 2012 there were 132,000 licensed massage therapists in the United States.[8] While adults generally know when, where, and why they need a massage for various aches, strains, and pains, I do not often come across pediatric patients who have had massage therapy. Research shows some beneficial health effects of massages in pre-term infants,[9,10] but in general, my experience with adult patients who have chronic pain shows that in patients who have had some manual therapy work, it takes a few more visits to get the results I expect.

NEUROCRANIAL RESTRUCTURING

Neurocranial restructuring, is a registered trademark of Dr. Dean Howell, a naturopath based in Washington, and combines deep muscle massage, craniopathy, Reiki, and Bilateral Nasal Specific Therapy, creating a treatment option intended to correct physiological imbalances caused by trauma, compression, and misalignment. This last therapy, Bilateral Nasal Specific Therapy, is a form of structural work that seeks to balance the symmetries in the face using a balloon inserted into the nostrils, which is then inflated.[11] Balloon dilation is used across the medical fields of cardiology, urology, ENT (ear, nose, throat), and neurosurgery, usually in a controlled operative setting; however, its use in outpatient pediatrics is uncommon.

Neurocranial restructuring is a very new approach, and so I would caution parents to carefully look into NCR before making their decision.

My first exposure to a patient that had experienced a procedure of neurocranial restructuring was in my pediatric office. The patient, a 3½-month-old infant, was there for a well-child exam. In reporting the history, the mother reported that at birth there were some latching issues for which the mother took the baby to receive neurocranial restructuring. She was very happy to report that after the first session the latching was no longer painful on her breast. She also stated that he had received a total of four sessions: two sessions a month for over 2 months. As I proceeded with the physical exam, I held on to his feet to start bicycling the legs. My usual procedure is to work up the legs, checking the range of motion and the tensions, eventually reaching the hips. I did not get past the knee. Like the flip of a switch, this calm, happy baby started to fuss and get red in the face. I stopped and I asked the mother, "What just happened?" The mother responded, "Oh, he just thinks that you are going to treat him." Naturally, I was dismayed. I stopped and waited until he calmed down, and once he let me check his hips, I proceeded. As he lay there, I noticed something strange about the angle at which he held his head. I was on his right side, and while he could have been turning his head to look at me, the turn had a slight tilt to it. I rotated him on the table, so that I was now on his left side, and sure enough, he did the same thing on that side. He had the same slight turn with the same slight tilt. At 4 months, babies should start to have neck and truncal control to be able to tolerate lying on their stomach and to rolling side to side, respectively. Before that ability develops, when you lay them down, they usually lay straight. I suspected some underlying neck tensions, probably previously in place, but not fully addressed. At this point, the cause is unknown—the best approach is conservative and I would observe how the infant structurally develops.

PART II

MECHANICAL DERANGEMENTS AND TRAUMATIC STRAIN

PART II: OVERVIEW

Well into adulthood, it is still possible to recover the patient's health, even if the patient suffered multiple complex combination injuries in their early life or even in their earliest formation. Recovery *is* possible; the problem is that most people (and their doctors) do not understand that injuries compound and, over time, alter how we function. When the patient crosses over the threshold into "dysfunction" they are diagnosed with a "disease" and given a corresponding medication. Life is hazardous enough; accidents and injuries *do* happen. Even the modern lifestyle, with its improved dental hygiene and surgical procedures, ends up inducing additional strains. Yet we insist on speaking of health in terms of medical diseases. Perhaps we should instead communicate our problems in osteopathic terms, that of "strain patterns." Traditional osteopathy offers a completely different perspective on health, a mechanical perspective unique in the history of medicine. Disease is a *process*, a deviation from health, initiated long ago by injury. Undoing the injury and correcting the patient from that path allows the body to balance and heal itself.

CHAPTER 5

Introduction to the Mechanical Body

W E A S humans are three dimensional creatures that have to operate upright against gravity. At any time during our lives when a trauma disrupts or displaces us in one dimension—usually resulting in some kind of bump or fall—we pick ourselves up, dust ourselves off and go back about our business. Most of us think that we recover from that little dust up. What I hope to explain in this chapter is that our mechanical body *adapts* that injury strain pattern. Tissue memory holds it in place and uses other peripheral tissues to balance it and to keep it in check. When it's just one small injury, a young body full of vitality can deal with the trauma, and maintain postural control over the strain, going about its daily routine *without feeling that injury at all.* But long after an injury has occurred, the memory of it remains in the tissue. That memory becomes hard wired into the messaging system of the brain and spinal cord. All of this happens right at the moment of impact. The injured tissue changes and *remains* altered; we osteopathic physicians can feel that dysfunctional tissue. In order for traditional osteopaths to accomplish seemingly impossible results, those traumatic memories need to be dug up and reduced so that the body's metaphorical inbox can be cleared of these old messages.

FORCE OF IMPACT

The impact on our bodies at the moment of injury can be described by a simple mathematical equation known as Newton's Second Law of Motion; namely, that force is equivalent to the mass of the object multiplied by its acceleration or deceleration, represented as $\mathbf{F} = \mathbf{m} \times \mathbf{a}$. It *would* be as simple as that, if we only existed in the angular square universe of Euclidean geometry. However, our structure is a bit more complex, and the way in which our living tissue deals with these forces is another complicated matter that cannot completely be described by a single formula. When I assess a patient, I look at the patient like a crime scene. Starting from the immediately obvious—that the patient has a functional and structural problem—osteopaths trace back the problem to the point in the past when they did not have the problem. Something happened in between those two points in time to disrupt the normal flow. The question then becomes, what violence has been perpetrated upon this body?

DIRECTION OF IMPACT

The direction of the impact upon our three dimensional physical body is critical in how we adapt the injury and function thereafter. When I assess a patient, I always ask about the mechanism of injury, that is, how did the injury happen, who witnessed the event, and so on, so that I can better understand the nature of the original injury. When I hear the story, I also examine the patient and feel for the vector of injury. Again, a vector is a force with direction; on the exam table, the patient's body will have the feel of being in motion, or a limb will feel like it is acting or moving on its own. When we lie still and are at rest (especially while we are asleep) all of our muscles should be inactive. The implication is that this is an injury pattern—something is making theses muscles and tissues act abnormally. Externally applied force is absorbed into living tissue. Young elastic tissues can absorb this force and contain it, controlling it by dispersing tensions throughout the body.

AGE OF THE PHYSICAL BODY
AT THE TIME OF INJURY

A fully mature physical body that sustains a simple vector injury can balance and "self-treat." For example, falling onto grass—which will have a smaller force of impact compared to cement because of the softer landing—and then getting up and dusting ourselves off (followed by walking around) usually has us feeling better. This is because the small force of impact puts an upward force into our tailbone. Walking and moving about frees up the sacroiliac joint, and gravity allows for a downward motion of the tailbone. The self-reduction of this simple injury can be explained by Newton's Third Law of Motion, that of equal and opposite reactions to any action. We are left fully pain free, unrestricted and functional when the gravitational drag on the sacrum and lumbar spine is equal to the compressive force of the fall. This is a fairly basic example of exercise and gravity as a therapeutic decompression force, precisely reducing a single traumatic vector.

Children and teens whose physical bodies are not yet mature have more difficulty dealing with traumatic injury. They appear unharmed, but that does not mean that they are not altered. In fact, they retain that injury pattern and mold their systems around it as they develop. While it may seem that the results of a child's maturation are purely from genetic inheritance, including their later susceptibility to injury or illness, all too often I see old injuries underlying current medical problems.

Injuries in infants and toddlers are insidiously devastating. Not yet fully formed, infants and toddlers are mostly water and soft tissue. The vector of injury is adapted by the watery tissue; it is embedded into the body and molded around during *development*. Shortly after an injury, parents think their children are fine, because their pediatrician examines them and finds nothing currently wrong. It is only later that the injury is manifested outwardly in the child's physical body as they try to grow. Often a parent will observe some asymmetry in their child's walk, or they'll compare the child's development to an older sibling and notice something different. They cannot express it, but feel as if something is not right. In the sections to follow, addressing specific osteopathic cases, I hope to share how to find clues in the physical body that will help parents identify where and how structural restrictions are acquired, and the best ways to unfold these tensions.

CHAPTER 6

High Velocity Injuries

W E ARE organic soft tissue wrapped around a bony framework of levers, gears, suspension cables, bridges, pulleys, and piston activity. Our bodies were not meant to be transported through space at high velocity. Even worse, we are not meant to suddenly decelerate. Recall the old saying: "It's not the fall that kills you, it's the sudden stop." Most high velocity injuries lead to a compressive load from impacts on the soft tissue. In the human body, these forces can be transmitted farther along to another part of the body, resulting in a local injury with a non-local source.

FALLS: GENERAL CONCEPTS

Of the types of injuries a child's body can sustain, one of the most devastating is a fall. Falls can be simple or complex. **Simple falls** are univectoral, in one forceful direction, and have a fairly simple treatment strategy. **Complex falls** are multi-vectoral and cannot be easily deduced. Each impact on each body part has a direction. Often, the order of the impacts cannot be recalled by the patient and so undoing each impact in the correct order can be impossible. As a result, the treatment strategy is not so simple. Each visit cannot be planned or predicted; when the patient comes in with a complaint, the osteopathic physician has to follow only what the tissue will allow for that day.

According to the Centers for Disease Control (CDC), 40 percent of all traumatic brain injuries between 2006 and 2010 were caused by falls. In children ages 0–14 years, 55 percent of traumatic brain injuries were caused by falls. In seniors over 65, the rate is at 81 percent.[12] Traumatic brain injury is diagnosed by examining to see if there is alteration of consciousness. These are significant injuries and the severity of the fall will usually bring the patient to the hospital for emergency treatment. The patient is altered at the time of impact. They continue to suffer the effects, a fact often unknown to the patient and those around them.

For general pediatricians, what we see most are minor falls onto tile or carpet from 3 feet or less. Most pediatricians give guidance to parents based on the immediate acute findings upon inspection of the child's body. As a traditional osteopathic physician and pediatrician, I give additional guidance to parents, instructing them to observe any behavioral changes, personality and sleep changes over the course of several weeks following even a minor fall.

Falls: Top to Bottom, Bottom to Top

The types of falls where the impact is perpendicular to the line of the body can have long-term effects depending on the height of the fall, and whether it occurs at the top of the head or directly to the bottom of the rear-end. These can occur as a direct impact to the tailbone or on the head. Direct impact due to a fall on the head deserves its own special attention as a subset in the category of traumatic brain injury, especially in adults or in children over 5 years old (well after the skull plates have closed and fused). Often, patients who survive landing upside down during a car accident and come to me for help were restrained by a seatbelt. Even though they do not have direct head impact, I always find the force of the accident to be in the head. In an infant, their heads mold to the impact. Over time, they mold the area of impact into the bones. While there is often a cosmetic issue, more importantly, the functional aspect of a child's development is directly affected. How trauma affects a child's function can vary depending on the area of impact. I often ask parents about sleep changes or behavioral changes.

Often, top-down impacts can cause chronic congestion problems, throat or tonsil infections, or lymph node infections. For example: Lindsay is a young woman who came to my office several times a year for lymph node infections in her neck. Despite the infections having been shown to be very responsive to antibiotics, on her fourth visit, I started to notice that something was wrong. I asked her to lie down for an exam looking for other lymph nodes, and as soon as her head was resting on the table, I noticed the veins in her neck pounding. I asked her if she had ever hit her head or been in a car accident. It turned out that several years before, while away at college, she was hit by a car while riding her bicycle. The car hit her from the side with such force that she flipped upside down and the top of her head hit the hood of the car. The pressure of having her head jammed into the car compressed her head down into her neck. The blood flow and tissues of her neck were now crammed downward, which explained the pounding. Her neck was literally a "bottleneck." As a result, her lymph nodes were sluggish and were poorly draining infections. I gave her another prescription and had her come back for an osteopathic treatment. Upon her return, a more in-depth medical history revealed migraines, neck pain and chronic knee pains, all of which were related to and caused by her accident from several years ago.

Most conventional doctors would not attribute the cause of chronic lymph node infections to an old trauma. Moreover, most would consider her multiple chronic medical problems *coincidental*. To the traditional osteopath, problems like these are all related and instigated by one traumatic cause. The osteopathic secret is to get the trauma out of all the tissues, from head to toe. Only then will all of her migraines, neck pain, knee pains, and even her chronic infections resolve. The secret is to "undo" the trauma.

Lindsay is now much improved. She doesn't get migraines anymore, and I rarely see her for lymph node infections. When she is stressed from work, she may experience a tolerable and treatable headache or a sinus infection, but this is the exception. She is also happy with the improvement of her acne and general state of her facial skin. She and I agree that she has not been "cured" of any of her problems. Her overall improvement attests to the understanding that a treated, mechanically unrestrained structure functions better and can better deal with inherent genetic tendencies.

Falls: Front to Back, Back to Front

Simple falls that I describe as being front to back can be belly forward or face planting (the difference between the two being the angle and location of impact). When our body flies forward, we fall at an angle which allows us time to control our fall and prevent our head from impact. The trade-off to preventing blunt head injury is that the neck whiplashes as we pull back. Patients who experience this may have long, prominent veins underneath the chin. In adolescents and adults, acne can result. In a forward face plant, there is no time to prevent facial impact. Facial impacts on infants and toddlers show up in the eyes and the area around the eyes. As they grow, the eyes may be more recessed back, dark circles under the eyes may appear, and there will be noticeable signs in the area between the bridge of the nose and inner corners of the eyes. The deeper recessed eyes may result from the force of the impact "pushing back" the eyes, as well as from the shock impeding the forward growth of the bones that form the eye socket.

Falls flat on one's back can cause several major areas of injury, namely to the pelvis and lower back, the back ribs, or the back of the head. Each tissue area may have varying disease presentations one week, one month, or one year later. The degree of tissue damage depends on the height from which the fall occurs, the terrain against which we fall, and our skeletal maturity at the time of the injury.

Falls: Side/Lateral Impacts

Side falls are always deceptive. In some cases, they may even be side *drops*. The only difference is the actor upon whom the action is directed. When kids fall on their side on their own, it is usually not as bad, because they are lower to the ground. Their height at the time of their fall mitigates the damage they would normally receive due to their not being fully formed. Side drops caused by another person are definitely worse. When a child is carried, they are usually carried by someone taller. The height at which they are dropped influences the force of impact their relatively younger bodies must absorb. When they are picked up, they *appear* unharmed, but they and their tissues are, in fact, altered—for life.

In a side fall, no bones are broken. The force of the fall is distributed over a larger area of the body, and the immature tissue has to absorb that force and shock. The child is seemingly fine, but when the muscles and bones start to grow, problems arise. In higher force impact falls or impacts at a younger age, the developing child will manifest musculoskeletal asymmetries. The impacted hip will be smaller; that leg may grow to equal the other non-impacted leg, but its function will be impaired. You can observe it in a person's gait: the hip will not be able to swing front to back and the leg will tend to swing in because the hip is jammed into the sacroiliac joint. Often in adulthood patients will complain of a "bad" side. Everything on one side has a problem, the arms and the legs, the neck, the face, and the jaw. The blood drainage system of the veins will be more prominent on that same "bad" side.

Christine is a prime example of the way in which a lateral side impact in childhood can have long-term effects, well into adulthood. She complained of chronic right-sided back and rib pain for years. The pains coincided with gaseous intestinal discomfort, causing loud burps. She would have to rub and massage her back to get the gas moving along before she could get relief. She also has varicose veins from her pregnancies, with the more painful ones being found on the right leg.

The right veins being more problematic was not coincidental. From my medical perspective, the most interesting feature on her face was a network of bluish veins that started at the right side of her neck. Many conventional doctors would not think much of these veins; certainly most would not see them as related to the varicose veins in her legs. I see it as a result of a right-sided drainage problem of the veins, whose congestion originated at the center of the right-sided back and rib area.

It turned out that when Christine was one year old, she was placed in a walker and somehow managed to scoot herself to the edge of a set of steps. She tumbled over three steps and fell onto her right side with the upper half of her body hanging over the hard inner rim of the walker. This history is not coincidental. The side impact of the walker into her infant ribs is not only contributory, but is rather *causative* of the current problems she suffers today. It took about eight visits before the facial veins would recede. Her back and rib pains are much better and, as a consequence, the gas and abdominal distention are not as bad. She rarely ever comes in anymore.

Complex Falls

Complex falls are the most difficult cases I treat in my practice. The reduction of each vector of impact can only be accomplished when the patient presents the problem and if we can assess them accurately. They have multiple pains and complaints. Falls down stairs are particularly devastating, and falls with head impact and tumbling are truly complex, and may lead to permanent disability. These cases are never easy, and patients often give up.

When a patient comes in with a complaint, it is because they have a pain they want treated. The most painful area in the body is usually an area with multiple tissue strain. The traditional osteopathic physician will address the "piled up" injuries in that area in order to free it up. But there is a limit to how much a body will allow in any one visit; after a point, the tissues will not release any further, at which point the body must be given time to recover. This is what makes complex falls so difficult: complex falls, with multiple vectors of injury, mean that we can only treat what and where the tissue will allow itself to be reduced. The vectors of injuries cannot be logically deduced, because they tend to have become tangled up and buried underneath, jumbled together with underlying, older injuries. Over time, the strain patterns settle and set in, like concrete.

Olga is 65, and was referred to me by her ENT (ear, nose, and throat) doctor for dizziness. One year ago, she fell down a flight of stairs. She lost consciousness, and only remembers her heel getting caught on a step before she tumbled. Her vertigo was so bad that she fell another four more times after her initial fall. Now, one year later, she is on disability due to a post-concussive syndrome. She has brain fog, she hurts all over, and she is dizzy all the time. The first time I evaluated her, I suspected that she had fallen on her left side and hit the back of her head on the left side. I *felt* a depression in the bony part of her skull on the left side behind her ear. I *sensed* a compressive force in that area, going from left to right. Every time she comes in, she is very bad, and each time I have a plan in my head for what I want to accomplish. But so far I had not accomplished anything other than helping her to feel a little better every time.

I started to suspect that the initial fall was the most traumatic, and I wanted to try to address it. She came in with severe back pain. She tried to straighten up her posture, and when I examined her, I found that she was in a twist. Her upper back was going left, and her lower back was going right. I spent the whole visit trying to figure out why she was so twisted. It turned out that she had a severe spasm in her diaphragm, and she responded well when I treated her sitting up. The lesson I take away from this case is to no longer try to plan out what *I* think she needs. Whatever tissue is in trouble when she comes in is what I address; this is my role as an osteopath.

Most high velocity falls and accidents result in multiple strains that lead to spinal instability later. In adults, surgery for spinal instability—from herniated discs, spinal stenosis, spondylosis, or spondylolisthesis—only locally addresses the decompensation. The surgical area scars up and impedes the balancing of tensions from more distant tissue. Children, and especially infants, who are mostly soft tissue and are still developing their bones, do not break, but rather bounce. As a result, the problems do not manifest until much, much later. In childhood, they may or may not show overt signs of restrictions in growth or development. They may even grow and develop with little to no apparent musculoskeletal problems... until later. Structurally, they may even appear to be symmetrical, but functionally, they are out of balance; their physiology is no longer "normal." They and their body are suffering.

For example: Rebecca first came to me as an adult woman after being referred by her neurologist for migraines (she also had fibromyalgia). Six years prior in her mid to late twenties, Rebecca entered the conventional medical system for breathing problems. Cardiac and pulmonary evaluation turned up no organic or structural cause. An MRI showed a small 5 mm cyst on her spinal cord in her thoracic region with some pooling of spinal fluid. She attributed all her symptoms to this cyst. A cyst anywhere on the body the size of a pencil eraser head would not be significant. But in the enclosed space of the nervous system, could it be just big enough to cause all these problems? She consulted a renowned specialist neurosurgeon, who felt that it was too small to cause all her symptoms.

However, at the age of 9, Rebecca had fallen down a flight of stairs, an old injury which served as the focus of our sessions. The first time I examined her head, it felt to me as if her skull was fractured into eight wedges, with all parts moving asynchronously. I was not surprised that she had migraines; her cranium wasn't functioning as one unit! Each part bobbed and weaved this way and that. This was my experience of the *motion of her brain and the overlying bones of her skull.* With her head in my hands, I applied a gentle, reassuring hold to secure and reduce the bounding and bobbing *feel* of the different pieces of skull. It took almost twenty minutes before she finally settled down.

In five treatment sessions with me, she reported that she felt no changes, and planned to stop our visits after her annual vacation with her fiancé. Even though I felt her tissue's tensions changing, and even though I felt as if I had accomplished something in settling down her body, I agreed that she should discontinue our sessions. She came back from vacation exclaiming that she and her fiancé had seen a huge change. She noticed that she could do 50 percent more work than before. She could carry more luggage. She could walk farther and for a longer period of time. She came back from vacation and resumed her osteopathic treatments. Since then, she and her now-husband have moved out of state to start their new life together, but she did ask me to recommend an osteopath (like me) to continue her treatments.

ROLLS

By far, one of the most common accidents in infancy is rolling injuries. Even at a low height, rolling can cause problems later in childhood. Rolling injuries induce a spiral strain on the soft tissue of the body from head to toe. That strain is locked in deeper if the impact is on a harder surface, that is, hardwood or tile floor. At the time of the rolling injury, most infants and children do not manifest problems; some even see it as a game. It is only much later during growth spurts that children will present with problems that may or may not be a musculoskeletal problem.

Think of a toy Slinky. Fresh out of the box, the Slinky is a large, loose spring: the coils stack nice and easy on top of each other and, when pulled on either end, they can open and close evenly at each level. A lightly used Slinky, with even one coil caught above or below, is not able to freely expand and lengthen. A heavily used Slinky, played with by multiple children, can have multiple coils caught at multiple levels. Stretching this garbled up Slinky will be difficult, and sometimes near impossible. Quite often, parents report a fall caused by rolling off the bed or couch, usually just before a diaper change. The bony vertebral column in the infant is still early cartilage, pre-bone and some bone. The soft tissues around the bones will later become stabilizing ligaments, tendons, intervertebral discs, and muscles. The fibers of these tissues run the length of the spinal column and also cross over. Taken together, I view the spinal column not as a tower of blocks stacked on top of each other, but rather a helical structure (very much like the Slinky).

Rolling injuries are also one of the most common injuries in young children. They frequently occur in the toddler period, during the transition from a crib to a child's bed.

Sometimes, rolling strains are intentionally induced as part of a game that children play at parties, at the park and in fairly "controlled" environments, like those of kid's gymnastics classes and indoor playgrounds. Unfortunately, whether accidental or induced, the physical body can be altered.

For example: Kathleen is my older daughter. When she was 18 months old, photos would show asymmetry in her lips as she spoke. When she started to speak more, I noticed a slight lisp. When she bumped her head, her tongue would dart out and pull over to the right. I took her to my colleagues, but no one was able to provide a satisfactory answer.

As she got older, it got worse. I resigned myself to the fact that I could not help my own child. Instead, I started training her to keep her tongue behind her teeth when speaking "s" words. Then I noticed that, while she was running and playing, her right foot would splay outward while the left foot ran straight. Was this a coincidence? Her tongue, right hip, and right foot veered right. Was this all part of the same pattern of injury?

One day, when she was about six, I decided to test my theory. I laid her down on my bed and had her gently roll to the left several times. She exclaimed, "Mommy, its better!" She started to make a game of it and stated, "This is just like the time I played with Maggie at the park." Maggie had been my daughter's babysitter between the ages of one to three.

It turned out that one side of the park was on an incline, and that she and Maggie had liked to roll down the side. Apparently, they played this game many times and without my knowledge.

I treat her periodically, and she now runs beautifully and symmetrically. She had patterned the rolling strain into her brain at such a young age that undoing it will be a long, slow process just to get the tongue back toward the middle. I have accepted the fact that this process of recovery will take several years (which is reasonable, considering she had adapted this pattern into her brain for 4 years). Gradually, we will be able to take advantage of her ability to grow to augment the treatments, expanding her mouth to provide more room for the base of her tongue.

After finding the source of her ailment, her treatment is now more certain, more precise, and each session yields more permanent results.

Other structural changes are also coming into play: previously, she did not have very prominent cheekbones, and her face seemed flat from the side. Her upper (maxillary) teeth previously looked narrowed and small; now, she seems to have more prominent cheekbones and her teeth and smile are wider. Her primary teeth grew in fairly straight. She lost two baby teeth, and one 6-year molar came in as normal. Interestingly, two of her new bottom incisor teeth are veered and angled in the same direction. The left lower jaw six-year molar is a bit angled, again in the same direction (to the right). I do not believe that the three crooked secondary teeth are the result of the expression of genes but rather the expression of rolling *forces*, because they were present at their *formation*.

Our most respected osteopathic teachers always remind us to thank our patients for teaching us, and Kathleen's case has many learning opportunities that may help distressed parents:

1. Several attempts were made to treat the lisp, to little effect. After failures, it is reasonable to wait; no harm is done with waiting.

2. When a strain is precisely reduced, there are multiple effects that are dramatic and longer lasting.

3. When a strain is precisely reduced, the system may be shocked and may require "balancing" to re-teach it what it *should* have known, to help it recognize the prior state of "normal" from which it was deranged.

Rolling and tumbling is a special example of a very complex fall. When infants and toddlers tumble, it may outwardly appear that they are no worse for wear. Inwardly, their whole body may seem stiff. The bones of the cranium will be dense and tight, and often they will have a large singular vein alongside one or both cheeks. Another possibility is a smaller network of small fine veins. It is best to undo these vectors in children while they are still young—as they grow, the linear growth stretches out the strain pattern, and any kinks or bends in the pattern can, over time, be straightened out.

BLUNT FORCE TRAUMA

In cases of blunt force trauma, external force is applied directly to a small, localized part of the body. The type of long-term effects I see in patients with blunt force trauma injuries depends on the object, its mass, the distance to impact, and the age of the patient at the time of injury. The force of the impact on the tissue is directly proportional to the mass of the object and its distance (if it is a falling object; if the object traveled across a distance, then it is considered a missile with a trajectory). Because the force of impact is not distributed across the whole body, but is primarily absorbed by one area, that one area can be severely affected. In fact, not only the tissue is affected, but the underlying bone changes its nature. The injured bone has a hard density feel to it, and it will feel almost as if a crater or depression has formed and molded into the area. The tissue area actually experiences a crush injury, and its function is impaired. This impediment is not necessarily permanent; the living tissue *can* instantaneously respond and revert to its original nature *if* a counterbalancing reduction force is provided.

Rachel's case is a prime example of calloused, injured bone instantaneously changing its nature. Rachel came to me complaining of migraines, and after examining her, I found a depression in her right shin. Touching it caused her pain; it turned out that a heavy, thrown object had hit her when she was in college. In the 15 years since, she has lived with a painful pothole in her leg. In five minutes of osteopathic treatment, the issues plaguing the bone and tissue area were resolved. The pothole was no more; it had lifted up and smoothed itself out, and no longer caused her pain in that area. Rachel still talks about it; we still both marvel at the instantaneous change. To this day, she tells me, "You did some sort of magic and it was healed immediately. It no longer feels like a bruise, and the visible indention is 90 percent gone."

MOTOR VEHICLE ACCIDENTS

The human body was never designed for high velocity movement through space, such as it experiences while traveling in a car. In fact, this state of forward movement of the body in space is so foreign to our body's tissues that impact and collision are not even necessary for the body to be permanently altered. I have reached a point in my practice where I believe that the force of a car accident, no matter how mild, is enough to impress damage into the body *forever*.

When I take an injury history, I ask patients to give me a play-by-play account of what happened, beginning several minutes before the impact. Where the accident took place is of primary importance: on city streets, velocity at the time of impact is much less than it would be on a freeway. What were the weather conditions? Was the road slippery? From what direction did the impact come? What types of cars or trucks collided? How did the patient's vehicle come to a stop? How damaged is the vehicle? Where is the damage on the vehicle? Was the patient rear-ended or T-boned? Was the patient restrained? Did the airbag deploy? Was there blunt force head trauma? Did the head impact the steering wheel, the side window, the windshield, or the headrest? If the patient was a passenger, what was she or he doing at the time, and how was their body positioned? Before coming to a stop, did the car swerve, spin, or flip?

The physical impact of a collision leads to structural compromise and soft tissue injury. The osteopathic physician can palpate the force of the impact on the tissue. The tissues change their nature by bearing the force and memory of the trauma. This information is very important; the force of the impact on the car also imparts a force onto the physical body, the evidence of which is in the *structure* of the tissue. When the car swerves, the momentum is also impressed in the fluid compartments of the body. When the car spins, the patient spins; there is a momentum that is indelibly impressed in the tissue and fluid compartments of the body. When the car flips, the whole body is distorted and disoriented in space. These fluid distortions in space, even without impact, may alter the body's structure, something that is evidenced in how the body *functions*.

An adult patient who survives swerving, spinning, and flipping will never forget the accident. They will say that their life was completely changed and disrupted the day of the accident. Their physical body carries a permanent scar and the physiologic memory of the trauma. The patient locks up the memory and stores it in the deepest recesses of the primitive animal brain. The reflexes of fear remain hardwired in the sympathetic nervous system. The patient may not even be consciously aware of these changes, as the patient remains in a state of "fight or flight" even at rest; they remain in what I call a "hyper-sympathetic" state. In adults, bowel functions may be altered, blood pressure changes can occur, and over time, hormonal changes may take place, as well as sleep disturbances and anxiety.

For the young, unformed infant or child body that experiences these high velocity forces, the effects are as serious as they are deceptive. Their young bodies mold these forces into their bone and tissues, the pathologies of which will take various forms later in life, depending on familial genetic tendencies as well as other previously and later acquired injuries. They may have sleep disturbances, autonomic nervous system imbalances and anxiety; the difference is, young children and infants will not have the words to describe these feelings of "not being right." They do not have the necessary sense of themselves to express these issues. In early childhood, the manifestations can vary from "disease" states to behavioral changes. As they grow up, their personality forms and can modulate and regulate their behavioral tendencies. By adulthood, with its accompanying skeletal and structural maturity, the trauma is still in place and contained, now regulated and balanced by tensions in the tissue. A body with these tissue tensions is, in effect, containing chaos, a chaos which will continue to drain the body's resources. The balanced mechanical system has to live, breathe, and move about in space against the effects of gravity; now it has an additional workload, that of contain-ing chaos. The body works harder than it should, and so ages faster than it would normally. At some point in the life of this aging mechanical system, when the reserves are exhausted, comes decompensation. The body can take it no more, resulting in exhaustion, pain, and disease.

According to the National Highway Traffic Safety Administration, there were about 5.6 million non-fatal car crashes in 2013 alone. However, the number of people reporting injury numbered only 2.3 million.[13] How many potential future patients with medical problems actually originated from a fender bender that wasn't reported because it was considered "minor?" How many little accidents, in which there is little to no bumper damage, are not reported—until the soft tissue injury manifests months or even years later? There are times in my practice when I feel that the vast majority of patients who come to me, having failed all forms of therapy, conventional or alternative, have an old car accident as the underlying cause of their condition. As with adults, the details of a car accident are important in treating infants and children. As I reduce the vectors of the accident strain pattern, their current symptoms often improve, even though that accident may have been months or even years old.

Rear-end Collisions

In rear-end collisions, the force of the impact is impressed into the immature bodies of infants and children. Outwardly, they don't appear affected at all; what happens at the time of impact is not visible to the eye. In children, the body and brain are mostly water. In adults, we know that soft tissue injury and whiplash can manifest several days, weeks, or even months later. Children, however, have pre-soft tissue; they are watery or gelatinous pre-form. What tissue whiplash can occur if they don't really have muscular form? In the language of osteopathic physicians, we say that infants and young children whiplash their fluid compartment. Their body and brain are shocked and jolted forward; even fluids obey Newton's First Law of Inertia. As the child grows, the tissues remain in this state of shock and forward displacement in space. Their posture and tensions are all out of balance, although different children will manifest this problem differently in their structure.

Ricky is a good example of the subtle manifestations of just one rear-end collision. Ricky's mother brought him in for chronic constipation. His bowel movements were only once weekly and he reportedly sat on the toilet for hours. He fell a lot as a child and rolled off the bed multiple times. I treated the muscles and tissues of his deep pelvis and his constipation improved. Bowel movements were now occurring every 3 days, and his mother was satisfied with the improvement. One day, while I was treating her for numbness and tingling in her fingers (from two old rear-end collisions), I asked how her son was doing. She responded that he was better but still constipated. She also remarked that he was sitting in the backseat in one of her rear-end collisions. I asked her to bring him in because I felt that he could improve on his bowel movements if I treated the car accident from his pelvis. It took two treatments, and within the same week, he started having bowel movements daily. I rarely ever see him anymore—only occasionally, when he has growing pains associated with growth spurts. He is a good (and easy) case of the "curative" return to health; not much has happened to his body, and not much has been done to him to cause difficulties in treatment or in recovery.

He is a simple case of how I attribute degree of causality. The multiple minor falls, rolls, and head injuries in early childhood contributed to 3 days' worth of constipation. The one rear-end collision caused 4 days' worth of constipation. By far, a car accident is worse (even though it occurred at an older age). Its higher velocity in the moment of impact contributes to a larger force of injury, greater than the sum of the impacts he accidentally caused to himself.

T-Bone Collisions

A side impact causes a side displacement of the physical body in space. Side impacts are one of the most deceptive types of collisions. Normally, the human body moves in a forward direction in space. Rear-end collisions propel the body forward, and the forward momentum is retained in the tissue memory as fluid inertia. It takes several small rear-end collisions for the sum total of the forward force and momentum to really affect development. By contrast, a single T-bone collision, no matter how small, is enough to alter the tensions in the body permanently.

For example: When I was 18 years old, I was T-boned in the parking lot of a mall. Although my passenger door was barely dented, when I look back to my college days, I had some minor bowel problems which I could not then explain. Throughout medical school and into my thirties, I did not rationalize my minor and occasional neck pains. My medical history past that point is short, compared to the majority of my patients—a wisdom tooth extraction, a surgery which required intubation for general anesthesia; a marriage with two childbirths, 17 months apart. Short though this list is, it is sufficient to cause unnecessary suffering. I only came to the understanding of my body after the realization that the car accident had been sitting in my body all this time. It has taken me one year of intermittent osteopathic treatments to get this car accident memory out of my body.

Complex High Velocity Swerving (with or without Collision)

Accidents resulting in complex high velocity injuries typically involve at least two directions of motion. Even without direct bodily impact and injury, patients are affected in the long term. Usually, the second direction comes into play when the wheels of the impacted automobile are directed right or left, while the force propels the car to swerve.

Annie is a patient with multiple sclerosis. She came into my office using the help of a walker. When she walks, her face and body are angled and veer to the right. Her "bad MS side" is "everything on the left." I believe this -sidedness in her MS stems from the complex car accident she was in when she was 10 years old. She was in the passenger side when her dad stopped at a stop sign to turn right. The body and tires of the car were already aimed to go right when they were impacted on the driver's side. They experienced the force of impact, after which the rightward acceleration occurred. Her left side is bad because that was the side that was hit more than 20 years ago. Over the course of a year and a half (and 30 visits), she has gone down two pant sizes and has been able to maintain her progress in physical therapy functional tests. One day, she told me that she had forgotten that when she was an infant, she and her mother were involved in a car accident. The rear-end collision was not minor: they were pushed forward and rode up onto the curb. My clinical experience with her leads me to conclude that two different high velocity injuries 9 years apart are significantly contributory, if not *causative,* of her later disease of multiple sclerosis. Other events in the course of her life contributed to the initial triggering and later exacerbations of her disease. She has failed acupuncture, chiropractic, and physical therapy. Prior to starting osteopathic treatments with me, she had gone from limping to a cane to a walker. So far, osteopathy has given her enough improvements to have hope and continue to move forward in her life.

Another possibility for swerving comes into play when the driver *overcorrects.* Swerving, even without impact, can have long-lasting effects on the physical body. I have many patients with bowel issues that I attribute to high velocity injuries. I treat them and their symptoms improve. I have to conclude that high velocity accidents that whiplash the intestines from side to side lead to symptoms of irritable bowel syndrome (IBS). These patients have gas, bloating, and diarrhea related to certain foods. The foods are specific to them and not always common culprits of food allergies. Blood allergy food testing is often negative, as is allergy skin testing. On the other hand, constipation can happen from an impact that causes the intestines to tighten up in a near twist (a true twist would cause an emergency blockage). If we view the intestines as a long hose that hangs down from the middle of our skull, and if that hose does not hang just right, then we have to ask: could the tiniest kink or tweak alter its function? The answer is a resounding yes.

Sasi is a fibromyalgia patient with two primary complaints: chronic muscle pain and IBS. She suffered daily on a pain scale of eight out of ten. It took weekly visits for 6 months to reduce her pain level to five. It took another 9 months of visits every two to 3 weeks to get her pain level down to three. She was very happy at a pain scale of three, and her life became easier. Thereafter, I saw her only intermittently, whenever her condition was really bad. I believe that I was able to help her once I attributed the cause of her muscular pain to the fall that her mother took down a flight of stairs while Sasi was 6 months in her mother's womb.

Through the course of 6 years we tried to address the IBS. At first we did the conventional approach: I tested her for food allergies which were negative. The only thing that helped her was specifically eliminating the items that she knew she could not handle. At each visit, while I am trying to figure out a patient's osteopathic mechanical causation of disease, we review their life over and over again.

It was only when I waxed philosophical about my suspicion of the terrible, life-altering and near permanence of high velocity car accidents that she told me about her non-collision incident. We had previously never discussed it because she assumed I meant *impacts* only. I tell my patients, "Every single little accident counts because these are not normal forces that a body is designed to endure." Two years prior to meeting me, she had spun out on a slick road. She did at least three revolutions before she slowed down and came to a stop. After hearing this, I worked to "un-spin" her intestines. Her immediate relief and near ecstasy response said it all. The feel of her distended bloated abdomen had changed instantaneously. It softened and started to gurgle, a sign that vegetative functions were returning. Thereafter, we continued this "un-spinning" treatment process from head to toe. She reports to me that her IBS is 60 percent better. She now only comes in when she needs to.

But the remaining 40 percent still bothered me. Several months later, during which time I had learned acupuncture, I called her in. I did an osteopathic treatment followed by a 26 needle acupuncture session. The next day, she brought her daughter in for an "un-spinning" osteopathic treatment because she was in the backseat the day of the accident. She reported to me that after our treatment that she had a normal formed stool for the first time in years. Several months later, her bowels continue to be normal and full. We are planning combined osteopathic and acupuncture treatments to eventually cure her.

The diagnosis and treatment procedure is similar in the case of an actual collision. JV was in the backseat next to his sister when they were both in a car accident, one month prior to the photos in Figure 1 (in the photo insert). During a high velocity swerve, his head hit the outside frame of his sister's car seat. In the photos, he was complaining of head and neck pain. Note the tilt of his head; he is an example of a complex injury: a high velocity force displacement and deceleration combined with blunt force trauma to the head. At his annual physical exam in July, his posture appeared affected. The belly was sticking out and the lower back seemed excessively arched. Patients injured in a car accident will experience back spasms and deep pelvic muscle spasms when in the seated flexed position. When they try to stand, they are unable to disengage that memory. The result is a tight backside and a more prominent belly.

CHAPTER 7

Low Velocity Injuries

IGH VELOCITY impacts can be described as the externally applied forces resulting from accidents that traumatize the body. In contrast, low velocity injuries can occur from as early as initial fetal development all the way through to delivery. In the lifetime of a human being's physical body, there are periods of risk for certain types of injury. The developmental period in the womb is rife with low velocity injury risks. The next period where low velocity injuries can occur is during the pre-teen period or teen period during procedural interventions (mostly dental).

Low velocity injuries in the womb occur in an environment of confinement and restriction. These injuries cause dull pressure pains, from which an organism would escape, if it could. Yet conventional primary care pediatricians and obstetricians do not even consider these types of injuries as playing a significant role in the developing bodies of fetuses and newborns. Even if the obstetrician is aware of the mechanical constraints upon the baby, there is very little that they can do. Their role is to care for the mother and help deliver a living newborn with as few complications as possible, given the particular medical condition of the mother. For osteopathic physicians, the fetal history and birth history play significant roles in the early years of a child. Speaking as a pediatrician, these low-force injuries may structurally shape a child well into adulthood and can even contribute to their personality.

COMPRESSIONS

Low-force compressive loads on the developing brain and body of the fetus in the womb can be caused by multiple maternal medical issues that affect the uterine environment. This is purely a matter of the fetus not having enough room in utero to grow.

Generalized compressive loading comes from pressure upon the fetus from all directions. This usually occurs in first pregnancies (when the maternal uterus has not yet been stretched by a prior pregnancy) and in cases where the mother has a prior history of pelvic trauma. But it can also occur in cases of multiple gestations, which can result in crowding of infants in utero. A traumatized maternal pelvis has enough difficulty with one baby; with twins or triplets, the maternal uterus may not be able to stretch far enough. Usually, one fetus bears more of the load; in multiple gestations of three fetuses or more, all the babies bear compressive loads on the head. If they have to be delivered prematurely, because the preemie body is primarily water and not yet fully formed tissue, gravity causes a further compressive drag on the fluids of the body. All preemie infants will have to deal with gravity at an earlier stage than planned.

A breech fetus in the last trimester experiences generalized compressive loading when there is little room for movement. The fetus's head is stuck under the maternal liver and as the fetus tries to grow and expand, it meets a counter compression force that translates down through to the fetal neck and upper middle back. Ideally, the immediate treatment would be for the fetus to turn by itself. Many methods and modalities have been offered and attempted to "induce" the baby to turn. The technical term is "manual version" which simply means turning the baby by use of the hands. That term implies both an external force and *coercion*. Breech babies may have problems with hip development, which general pediatricians check at each visit. But a breech baby that has *not* turned after multiple attempts from an external force is usually in far worse shape than if no attempts had been made at all. Many end up being the loudest and fussiest babies, more so than if they had been left alone. The maternal instinct in response to their infant's screams is correct—those *are* screams of pain. These babies have headache. There are several studies that look at the colicky screaming infant, two using the specific pitch of the cry as an indication of colic,[14, 15] one case report regarding a neurologist's concern about headache,[16] and another report linking migraines with colic.[17]

This is because babies who are breech and left alone until a delivery by C-section have only the downward compression vector on the head and body. I find that babies that have tried to turn by themselves have twisting and turning tension strains in their face, head and neck. Babies that have had doctors or midwives attempt a turning, whether successful or unsuccessful, usually have multiple strains of greater complexity. This is because a fetus trying to turn itself will stop on its own once tensions *start or increase*. However, an external set of hands would require a higher amount of tension and restriction (to register a higher threshold of force) before terminating the procedure. I believe that the best way to address breech fetuses is traditional osteopathy. We remove (by reducing) prior traumatic vectors of injury in the maternal pelvis, which releases muscle spasms, which allows muscle relaxation, which allows uterine, back, and pelvic stretching. The fetus senses the new freedom and moves toward that freedom *on its own*. I have several patients who tell me that their baby turned later in the week following a treatment for back pain or excessive swelling. The second best way of addressing a breech fetus is simply to plan for a C-section.

Babies who are large for their gestational age, with or without maternal gestational diabetes, will experience the same kind of compressive loads, only more uniformly across the whole body. The treatment for them is simple: birth. Obstetricians generally have a sense when a large baby may be too risky to attempt a vaginal delivery. It is at this point that they may come to an agreement with the mother to schedule a C-section. These infants and children generally do well on their own because growth itself is a therapeutic treatment. If they do have problems, they usually appear to have a local area of restriction and strain. Without any other traumatic injuries, they are not difficult to treat osteopathically.

Localized compressive loading or pressure on a body part of the fetus will lead to problems specific to that area. The pre-pregnant maternal pelvis may have a soft tissue tumor, a fibroid, cyst, or myoma, which could grow and compete with the fetus for space. If a limb or body part is wedged or trapped and is not free to move, blood flow is impaired as the tissue attempts growth and development. How these localized tissue injuries manifest can vary: in the limbs, there may be a gross deformation, with an orthopedic diagnosis or none at all. Those who do not appear to have visible structural problems may have functional problems with their gait or growing pains later in childhood. In the head, trunk, or body, growth itself can be therapeutic, as it allows for tissue expansion in all directions. Physical evaluation should reveal a local area of tissue restriction. Traditional osteopathic treatment should be localized, and the patient is expected to respond almost immediately.

SHEARS

Elastic tissue that is stretched so far that it has problems returning to its resting length (i.e., it is too stretched out and slacked) is described as **sheared**. A traumatic shear injury happens when tissue is stretched beyond the normal physiologic range. A common shearing injury I see in adults who complain of back or neck pain is one that is acquired while missing the step off of a curb or accidentally stepping into a pothole or depression. The step down is not anticipated and the hip joint is pulled downward and out. It feels "loose" and unstable. In the upper body, another tissue area that can be sheared out is the shoulder joint. Many people can understand being pulled by a large dog on a short leash. That sudden jolt from the animal pulls the arm out of the shoulder socket and the shoulder does not feel right.

Shears in infancy primarily occur during the birth process. All babies experience a limited amount of shear as they are compressed and hyperextend their heads, neck, and upper back as they exit the birth canal. Additional extraneous shearing forces can be imparted upon the head and neck of infants when they become stuck, and the obstetrician needs to get the baby out. Forceps are still used in difficult deliveries to guide the infant out the birth canal. Forceps placed along the sides of the cheeks cause the face to experience compression, and pulling the baby down can impart a traction or shearing strain on the head and neck. When a single baby or even multiples are stuck, and a C-section has to be done, the minimal shear is generally not as consequential, so long as they are pulled out by the buttocks. Vacuums are now more commonly used to extract a stuck fetal head, as the vacuum does not cause as much a compressive force on the cheeks and face of the infant as compared to forceps. The trade-off is a shearing strain that starts from the upper middle back and continues all the way up through the infant brain.

Shears also can also be imparted on other parts of the body. The limbs are vulnerable to shearing, when an infant, toddler, or child is pulled. In a C-section, if the infant is grabbed by the shoulder or hip and traction is placed to pull the baby out, a mild shear may be induced.

In general, shears are easier to treat than compressions. Shears only require a steady hand and a broad application of the palms of the hand. In effect, the treatment of a shear is a gentle compression. A compression injury, however, is always more difficult to undo. The treatment for a compression injury is *decompression*. Some of our most basic techniques of decompression, however gentle, can *cause* a shear if it is inappropriately applied. Osteopathically, if overtreatment occurs and a patient reacts negatively, it is always possible to correct an overcorrection.

Gravity

We all know gravity as the physical force that keeps us anchored to the ground. It is the force that causes us to fall, and is what makes our face drag and sag as we age. It is the force that drops our breasts, belly, and buttocks over time. Gravity as a force is dependent on the height of the object and its weight. Think of the added weight of a pregnant belly. Now, consider that during the 10 months of pregnancy, the increasing weight load is causing a downward shear, a very special form of a repetitive stress injury. Now consider a normal fetus in an uncomplicated pregnancy where the head is down. The developing fetal head is experiencing a gravitational downward shear. Now consider a non-ideal pregnancy, such as a breech positioning, where there is a downward compression, circumferential compression, and downward shear. Now, consider other pregnancy complications having an additive effect. Gravity is a special type of chronic repetitive stress injury. Often, gravity is used as a treatment to balance their strain, as a therapy. In infants, the treatment is used by holding the baby upright, as a cure for fussiness or reflux.

Twists and Torsions

Fetal movements and in utero gyrations happen within a very narrow range within a constricted space. If the baby does this on his or her own, it is within his or her own physiologic normal. Twisting strains do happen (to a lesser degree) as a normal process of birth. In planned C-sections or an uncomplicated vaginal delivery, these minor twisting strains are minimal and infants can, eventually and over time, outgrow it. Pathological twists and spiraling torsions usually occur in conjunction with other strain injuries. This happens when the infant head is very stuck, and there is risk to mother or infant, or both. It is part of a desperate act and happens fast. In these emergency situations, it is not uncommon to have compression, shearing and torsion upon the infant's head and neck, all in a quick moment in time. The obstetrician will choose either forceps or a vacuum to extract a stuck baby. The twist alone is usually within the normal range of motion for a fetal head and neck. But repeatedly twisting the head and neck while having forceps compression on the infant's cheeks and hyperextending the neck, impart multiple vector strains, all in a matter of seconds to minutes.

This moment in time in the history of a patient's body can have a long term, daily effect lasting well throughout a lifetime.

I occasionally see adult patients with migraines or chronic neck pain with this type of birth history. The compression remains in their cheekbones, with the more severe tissue restriction occurring at the back of the head and neck. This is never an easy area to treat. It usually takes multiple visits. It is better to address issues like this in infancy, because once the tissue is free of restriction, growth and development is as near to unimpeded as possible.

CHAPTER 8

Repetitive Low-Force Stress Injuries

T HESE TYPES of strains happen slowly, and over a period of time, the effects become additive. Even in the case of a few slow, intermittent events of low-force stress, a fetus, infant, or child still may not fully outgrow the trauma. Most of the traumatic events that happen to the physical body affect us as three-dimensional structures. Undoing the traumatic vectors of a three-dimensional jigsaw puzzle is difficult enough; when it sets in place, as it does in an unformed, incomplete structure, undoing it is even more difficult.

MATERNAL FORCES AND REPETITIVE LOW-FORCE STRESS INJURIES IN FETUSES

Most pediatricians, obstetricians and family practice doctors are not aware of how repetitive low-force fetal injuries play out in the health of a human being. The first question that must be asked is what kinds of fetal injuries can possibly happen in the protected environment of the womb?

The most common structural impediment to the growth of a fetus, generally or locally, is one of positional compression or entrapment. These can be generally recognized by conventional doctors when the results manifest in a limb. We'll be discussing the less obvious implications of various types of fetal injuries.

The ideal state in the womb is one of calm. In the enclosed space, there is amniotic fluid to allow less friction in movements and to cushion the baby. Yet even with this cushion, external forces can influence the development of the infant.

Morning Sickness

"Morning sickness" is nausea (with or without vomiting) at any time during pregnancy. I find it unfortunate that morning sickness is considered normal; it is *not* normal for a pregnant woman to be made ill by her fetus. Worse still is the concept that a baby makes the mother so ill that she vomits. That this is commonly accepted by people, including the doctors of the conventional medical system, is wrong. Traditional osteopathy informs me that morning sickness is a result of the maternal vessel, the uterus, not adapting well to the hormones, the fluid load and stretch. I would suspect that prior to pregnancy, the maternal mechanical system experienced trauma.

If vomiting is severe, a condition called hyperemesis gravidarum, conventional concerns will include the hydration status of the mother and the fetus. Mechanically, the concern is that the repetitive compressive loading of the maternal diaphragm upon the uterus during vomiting will transmit force through to the developing tissues of the infant. If the position of the fetus is head down, the compression forces upon the baby are more significant, from buttocks through the spine into the head. If the baby is stuck and lying on the side, in a transverse position, the diaphragm pushes down on one side. If the baby's head is on the maternal right side and facing front, then compressive loading from vomiting affects the baby's left side. If the baby lies with the head on the maternal left side and facing front, then compressive loading will affect the baby's right side. If the baby is breech and vomiting is frequent, then the fetus has to deal with not only the maternal liver against its head while it is trying to grow, but also the intermittent compression of the diaphragm pressing on the liver, which in turn presses on the uterus. Newborn babies with this prenatal history often have problems nursing and are usually fussy. While they will typically outgrow the fussiness, if left untreated, the compressed tissues may manifest in toddlerhood in different and varying forms.

For example: A toddler was brought to my practice by her parents for consultation. At 18 months, well after she had learned to walk, the toddler had started to trip and fall. They described her legs as buckling and causing her to fall to her knees. They brought her to urgent care, the conventional approach of which is to evaluate for a hip or knee infection. The doctor referred her to me for a traditional osteopathic evaluation and treatment of a nonspecific musculoskeletal problem with her gait. In evaluating her ankles, knees, and hips, there seemed to be very little tension or problems of range of motion. Her prenatal history, however, was positive for maternal vomiting: twice weekly, from the fifth to eighth month of pregnancy. That is a *lot* of compressive loading upon the fetal head and body. After she was born, she was fussy, and nursing was difficult for the first 3 months. Her treatment was mostly cranial osteopathy to unload the compressive forces of the maternal vomiting. The results were immediate. We stood her up and she walked better. She only needed the one treatment. On a 6-month follow-up, the mom called and asked if she should come in for another visit. I asked if she was tripping and falling. The answer was no. Were there any other medical issues? The answer was no. Then she did not need to come in, I told her.

This case is complex, both in its history and evolution. The toddler's problem at 18 months was prenatally caused, and its causation was much older than her chronologic age; in fact, it was 21 months old. That it took one-and-a-half years before the fetal head injury manifested ill effects is one reason why the cause would not be considered by conventional pediatricians or pediatric orthopedic specialists. Mechanically speaking, vomiting imparts a univectoral load. It is simple, in that the force and loading occurs in one direction.

Braxton-Hicks Contractions

A more complex maternal force, one that plays a significant role in the first year of an infant's life, is that of Braxton-Hicks contractions. These are uterine contractions that occur before the infant is due. Considered "false labor," this term is so benign that it hides the insidious nature of the slow, repetitive compressive loading of the infant. These babies scream as they try to outgrow their traumatic history. Each contraction propels the fetal head and body down toward a birth canal that is not yet ready. The fetus is essentially forced into the role of a battering ram against a closed door. These newborns are in pain, causing their parents to instinctually fear the worst case scenario. They are convinced their child is gravely ill, but upon reaching the emergency room, they are told to let their baby cry it out, that there is nothing to be done. They are sent home without much help and with plenty of dissatisfaction and distrust that continues on past the colic period.[18]

Each contraction is, in effect, a *head injury*. Each contraction causes a direct compression from the top of the head all the way down to the middle of the upper back. I believe the crying and screaming is from *headache*. These babies are what I call "pacifier hungry." They will appear ravenous, sucking on anything proffered furiously; their urge and demand for it is just that excessive. This is because they are using the muscles of their face, mouth, and tongue to try to cause decompression.

New parents Greg and Michelle bring in their newborn, along with a report of Braxton-Hicks contractions having occurred throughout the last month of pregnancy. I am concerned and warn them that the baby may become "colicky." Sure enough, their daughter has more wakeful periods, during which she fusses and cries: she is just not a very happy baby. The effects of our first osteopathic treatment only last 3 days; after they left the office, the baby fussed less, nursed more easily, and slept better. She initially needed weekly visits (for 6 weeks) until we could all see that she was consistently getting better and *staying* better for a longer period of time. By 9 months I hardly ever needed to see her except for well-baby checks. Her mother now knows to bring her in when she becomes clingy, has decreased appetite, or inconsistent sleep schedule, which are all manifestations of an attempt to have a growth spurt. How do we know this? Because immediately after one treatment, she slept better, was less clingy, ate more, and then had a growth spurt. By 18 months of age, when she hurts she tells her mom, "*Owwie*. Doctor. Bye-bye."

DENTAL TRAUMA AND BRACES

Dental procedures and the repetitive nature of positioning the head and neck in the dental chair are some of the most difficult strains to reduce. This strain injury, although low velocity, is as permanent as any car accident. It is locked in *forever*, unless there is a matching external force to reduce it in precisely the manner by which it was induced. I consider it the second most insidious strain injury that is procedurally caused.

Sitting in a dental chair is an unnatural position. Nowhere in nature do we find the human body positioned in this manner. The muscles of the face and mouth are stretched out to an extreme; the head is positioned back and braced against a padded headrest (which causes the bones in the back of the skull to jam up); and the neck is stretched, arched up, and forward. The upward shearing strain pattern affects what I call the dental shoulder, the dental chest, and the dental hip. In an osteopathic treatment to precisely reduce dental trauma, I instruct patients to do a pre-treatment test by breathing in through their nose, and taking a deep breath. Most patients are unaware that their breathing pattern has been affected by what I call the dental brain, the dental face, the dental neck, the dental shoulder, the dental chest (and ribs), and the dental hip. At each body area, I engage and then disengage the memory of the dental strain pattern. I usually treat one side first, and then ask patients to do the test breathing again. This maneuver is 100 percent effective. Although patients believe that their breathing is fine, after I treat one side they can tell that their breathing has improved and ask that I treat the remaining side.

The next time your child undergoes a dental procedure, especially under sedation, please watch how the dentist and anesthesiologist position the head, mouth, neck, jaw, and shoulders. It would be even better to record the event in order to document it for use in osteopathic sessions. Observe the length of time during which your child is oddly positioned. Under anesthesia, the brain and spinal cord are asleep. The small, fine and deep muscles of these tissue areas are, essentially, trained to be in this position. Once the anesthesia wears off and the brain and spinal cord wake up, the strain pattern is accepted, adopted, and adapted as the "new" resting length, the "new" normal.

The body is lying down, at rest, with no gravitational forces to engage the postural muscles. Yet the head remains hyperextended on the neck. The neck is sheared upward, superiorly. The shearing tension pulls up on the shoulders, the chest, and the ribs. Meanwhile, the arms are down, which roll the shoulders and are positioned while being relatively flexed. The upward shearing effect can reach as low as the low back and hips. When I treat patients, I show them the effects of the dental injury patterns, which I refer to as the dental brain, the dental neck, the dental shoulders, the dental chest, and the dental hip.

Imagine this strain pattern, impressed into the body multiple times, attempting to stand upright against gravity. Every body part, from the top of the head to the tailbone, is sheared upward. The "wrongness" and desynchronized nature of this occurs when the arms hang down and drag the shoulders down into further relative flexion, while the structures above and below are stuck in extension or hyperextension. More asynchrony occurs at the pelvis; while truncal weight loads are supposed to be borne upon the pelvic bones, this cannot be done properly by the upward shearing nature of the dental strain pattern.

Dental bracing is a special nightmare in and of itself. Some orthodontists pull teeth to make room. I have patients who recall their sense of vulnerability and fear during dental extractions. Some plan the braces in stages, with the more humane way being preceded by a dental appliance that spreads the palate. Once the wires are placed, regular follow-up visits are usually short, and are for the purpose of tightening the wires.

Even though they are short visits, the head and neck position repeated often is, in effect, a repetitive stress injury. Most braces are placed for extended periods of time, usually between 1 and 3 years. I am especially disturbed when hearing reports that some begin the bracing process as early as 8 years of age.

With the increasing exposure of children to processed foods, snacks, and juices, more and more children are requiring dental cleanings, fillings, and crowns at earlier ages. Alterations in the tensions of the muscles in the head, neck, face, jaw, and shoulders of children are induced, while parents and patients remain unaware of the long-term effects and later contributions to musculoskeletal problems.

CERVICAL COLLARS

In dire emergency medical situations, we want to make sure the patient is breathing. We want to check the airway and make sure it is not obstructed. At accident scenes, we want to control the airway. We want to stabilize it, and work to position the head and neck in order to keep the airway clear and so as to maintain breathing. Paramedics put on a rigid plastic cervical collar to maintain the head and neck relationship, in case there are hidden fractures in the cervical spine. The accident victim must then be safely transported to a trauma center. All told, an accident victim may be stuck in a cervical collar for 6–8 hours. Not only are they still in shock and hyper sympathetic, remaining in that "fight-or-flight" mode, but they are now also in hyperextension. This is not a memory of trauma that they will escape easily, if they ever escape it at all. Without osteopathic treatment, this trauma is indelibly impressed in the deep, long-term memory of the brain and hard wired into the muscles. Most adult patients who go through this experience have problems with anxiety and sleep disorders when the neck is hyper extended. In a young infant or child, they go through all of this as well, but they grow up adapting all this strain and stress. It becomes a part of them; they have a hard time describing what they are feeling because most of the pathology is now a part of them.

INTUBATIONS (FOR GENERAL SURGERY)

I consider intubations to be among the most harmful procedures of those that cause repetitive stress injuries. Intubation plays an enormously unrecognized role in musculoskeletal injury and "disease" in later life. Early on in my journey studying traditional osteopathy, there were difficult cases, cases where I failed to help the patient recover. To improve my assessment abilities and my quality of treatment, I had to take an honest look at why I had failed to help these complex cases. My mentor clued me in to the dangers of intubations, and my eventual discoveries regarding the damage that this routine procedure can cause need to be made known to the general public, not to mention the future osteopathic physicians who must try to reduce the vectors of strain imprinted and conditioned into these now-altered resting muscle tensions after intubation.

In preparing for a surgery, the first step before administering heavy duty anesthetics is accessing and controlling the patient's airway. This is accomplished by putting an endotracheal tube (a firm plastic tube whose diameter is equivalent to a large drum stick) down the patient's airway. In and of itself, the tube only mildly irritates the airway; it is the external application of force to position the head and neck by others that negatively affects the relationships of the muscles in the face, head, neck, jaw, shoulders, chest, and the rest of the lower spine and hips.

In reducing the combined traumatic vectors of upward shearing and hyperextension, I try to educate my patients on what I call the intubated brain, the intubated jaw and neck, the intubated chest, the intubated shoulder, the intubated hip—the specific injury patterns that result from intubation. Most conventional doctors would not believe that intubation has long-term effects on the shoulder, lower back, and hips; however, in my sessions with patients who have been intubated, I proceed to treat the head, neck, jaw, shoulder, chest, back, and hip (most often the left). The traumatic vectors of intubation are nearly identical to dental traumatic strain patterns. My treatment of any patient who has had a past intubation involves engaging the tissues in their strain patterns, and then disengaging them. Patients can then compare the tensions, and feel for themselves how the reduction has improved their range of motion or breathing. I educate all my patients in this way; that way they know to come in after they have procedures done, so that I can undo the strain.

In infants and children, intubation is the most difficult low-force stress injury to reduce and re-train. The bones in the neck of the new-born do not start out as small, individual, whole neck bones. The new-born neck bone is made of three small pieces that grow, join, and then fuse together, usually at ages three, five, and seven.[19] Any high velocity or slow repetitive stress trauma, whether accidental or intentional, will alter the tensions of the pre-tissue and the relationships of those osseous centers, thereby affecting development. My specific osteopathic treatment for infants and children 5 years of age and under is a bit different. In adults, I am able to make use of their cooperation and time their muscular contractions at my direction. Children, who cannot cooperate in this way, require a different approach; in my case, a treatment involving specific finger placements and precise engaging/disengaging of their strain patterns. Different osteopaths will treat these types of injuries in children in different ways, but each follows this basic format.

PILLOWS AND SLEEP POSITIONING

When I was a medical student rotating in the emergency room of a big New Jersey hospital, I came upon an issue that continues to occupy my thoughts to this day. It was busy, as all big city hospitals tend to be, and there was an elderly gentleman to whom I had been assigned. He was in his seventies, and his blood pressure was high. While he was waiting to be seen, he was visibly uncomfortable on the gurney. His head, neck, and upper back were so stiff that he asked for a pillow. Now, if you have ever been in a busy emergency room, you'll know that clean pillows are a high value commodity. I ran around searching for one so that he could be comfortable. He absolutely needed it; he was so stiff that there was no way he could slump and relax, to flexibly mold to the flatness of the upright gurney. I realized that his head, neck, and upper back were *dependent* on a pillow to support him. There are worse things in life to be dependent on, certainly—for example, prescription or recreational drugs, alcohol, sex, even shopping—but it still represented a dependency, one that was currently crippling him. The memory of this case is still with me 20 years later, because his posture was fundamentally *wrong*. The question is, did the pillow cause the problem, or was it *evidence* of a problem?

Fast forward 6 years later: I am on call in an NICU, a neonatal intensive care unit. The night nurse did not know why, but one of the babies in her care was experiencing a drop in its oxygenation level, causing the alarm to sound. I checked the baby and realized that the nurse had left the baby on its back, placing a little folded blanket underneath the head to support the soft newborn skull. The problem was, it was too much: it positioned the baby's head flexed forward, causing the chin to tuck and kink the smaller newborn airway. I took the makeshift pillow away and the baby's oxygen level picked up. In exchange for easy oxygenation, we had to accept a more extended head and neck, as well as a flatter back of the head.

Most infant and newborn bedding does not include a pillow, and any pillows purchased in sets for infant bedding should be considered purely for decoration. It is only later in development of an older child or adolescent that I will see pillows influencing postural development. It may not be a causative agent in musculoskeletal problems, but it certainly does play a role in maintaining an injurious cervical strain pattern. It may be necessary to support the intubated or dental neck strain. In itself, by supporting the pattern, it causes the patient to invest in it further, locking in the injury. For this reason, it can be considered as being its *own* repetitive stress injury.

Based on my clinical experience, I teach patients that the purpose of a pillow is to support the *head*—not the neck. The normal curve in the neck (cervical lordosis) may become exaggerated if a pillow is too large. In a cervical lordosis, the back tissues at the back of the head and the top of the neck are shortened and tight. Having this neck tension

in place is uncomfortable and makes it difficult to rest, muc
Most people will pull the pillow all the way down to the sh
support all these structures and reduce tensions. The proble
the shortened tissue resting length is maintained throughout th   ...
They do not get a chance to stretch and gently lengthen. At night, when
sleeping on the back, a pillow used strictly to support the head allows
gravity to slowly and safely stretch the back tissues of the neck. I usually
instruct my patients to position the edge of the pillow just at the level of
the ears. I have also devised a few gentle, easy exercises for my patients
(included in the last chapter of this book).

Sleep positioning is as important in the pediatric structure as it is
in adults. In either group, it hints of tensions in ligaments, tendons, and
muscles of the backside. We toss and turn, trying to find a comfortable
position. The position we find comfortable invariably reduces our tension so that we can fall asleep. Falling asleep in that reduced tension
state—with shortened muscular length—allows the brain and spinal
cord to adapt and reset that shorter length as *normal.* Any activity in
daily life that stretches this new pathological "normal" is now seen to
induce a strain.

In children, belly sleeping is an indicator of a tighter backside, and
is very much a chicken/egg conundrum. Is the child so restricted that
arching the lower back reduces tension? Or does sleeping on the belly
originate as a good stretch to treat the 10 months of fetal flexion position that, over time, turns into a problem of having a lower back that
is too arched? In either case, once belly sleeping becomes habitual, it is
now a vicious cycle that feeds into itself. If belly sleeping continues well
into adulthood, it usually signifies deep tensions in the head, neck, or
lower back.

CHAPTER 9

━━━━━━━━━━

Combination Injuries

C OMBINATION INJURIES involve multiple simultaneous vectors on the body, and result in multiple types of injuries. The complex nature of these injury patterns is difficult to undo. The patient is treatable; it just takes longer and requires a slower, more thoughtful approach over a longer period of time.

SPORTS INJURIES

Exercise and play are both important in the musculoskeletal development of a child. It is therapeutic, as well as being good for stimulating bone growth while improving cardiovascular, respiratory and mental health. According to Stanford Children's Hospital, every year 30 million children participate in organized sports, and 3.5 million are injured (mostly with sprains and strains).[20]

Children participate in both contact and noncontact sports. The former, as most parents understand, can cause significant high velocity impact trauma, ranging from mild to severe. However, in organized sports, where there is a visible commitment to player safety, most parents assume there is little to no possibility of inducing a low-force repetitive stress injury into the body of a developing child that will alter, mold, and permanently change that body. The sports that are most likely to contribute to significant alterations in the musculature of a child are what I call "asymmetric sports." These are activities where one side predominates; as the spine attempts to grow and elongate, there are generally rotational constraints on the child. Some of these activities include swimming, basketball, golf, and soccer, just to name a few. Kids who swim have a tendency to breathe to one side. If they start early, at 5 or 6 years of age (well before skeletal maturity) the body can mold to that repetitive stress. The swimmer who constantly turns to breathe on the right side will chronically induce a rotation to the right in their neck and chest. When their body attempts to grow, not only will they have a difficult time turning left, but the chest wall enclosing the heart and lungs will have a difficult time expanding and elongating. Basketball has the same effect. The dominant hand will be the shooting hand, and that shoulder will always be higher, that side more stretched. There will also be some chest and truncal rotation to the other side.

In children who start young, both swimmers and basketball players can develop early scoliosis, with or without chest pain (although children who manifest these types of injuries are more likely to have underlying, previously acquired structural strains). Kids who start asymmetric sports while they are young mold a twisting, rotational pattern right through the middle of their chest. It is very plainly visible, and parents are very scared for their children when they hear complaints of chest pain. After reassuring them that it is not a problem with their heart, I have the parents stand right behind me while I point out the unequal shoulders, the curve in the back, the rotation in the back ribs, the twist in the hips, the stance, and feet placement. Without even touching them, I have the child pretend to do the activity and go through the motions in the opposite direction, using the other side. I have them repeat to a count of ten or so. The parents and I then recheck and we instantly notice significant improvement of all the parameters: the shoulders are more level, rib rotation is lessened, rotation of the pelvis is improved and feet placement is more equal.

COMBINATION MATERNAL AND FETAL INJURIES

When a woman is pregnant with her baby, she has to adapt to an increasing center of gravity several inches in front of her normal center of gravity (just in front of her lower spine). She has to learn to walk with an increasing pelvic weight load, and she has to accommodate a growing baby trying to stretch her uterus. Imagine a maternal pelvis that was previously injured from a high velocity car accident several years ago, one that still causes occasional back pain. We now have a strained uterus that does not stretch well against a growing baby, and is chronically tight upon the baby. The mother then develops vomiting, which further compresses on the baby. Now, imagine a high velocity accident occurring under these circumstances. While the fetus was supposed to be floating freely in an accommodating uterus, their mother falls down a flight of stairs, or her dress gets caught on a heel and she does a belly flop onto grass, or she is involved in a car accident. These babies will have chronic medical problems, going forward. The medical problems may be different from one another, but the causes are universally old, and sometimes decompensate with a new acute destabilizing injury. These cases take a long time to treat and are close to impossible to fully resolve. The only hope is to help the child's body free up when it tries to expand and grow over time; most pediatric patients do well with multiple visits over a period of time. In more complex cases and with an adult with early childhood strains, a span of years may be needed.

CHAPTER 10

Derailment and Recovery

T O THE traditional osteopathic physician, the beauty that unfolds in the safety of the amniotic sac as genes express themselves is by *design.* Yet this unfolding of a "plan of perfection" may be disrupted. Life is hazardous, and anything can happen at any time. Even the maternal uterus may pose some restrictions, limitations, and even hazards to the events unfolding within. The unbalanced, mechanically inefficient, and traumatized mother may be at risk for further external events and forces. So, the beauty and design of a life may have primary, secondary, tertiary, and even quaternary degrees of derailment from this perfection within.

Here, too, the philosophical contrast between conventional medicine and traditional osteopathy is significant. In conventional medicine, imperfect or altered genes lead to the expression of a disease. To scientists of the conventional medical system, defective genes are just... *there*; they coexist with normal genes. To them, these are just random derangements. To traditional osteopaths, there are forces early on in our formation that may be *causal* to that imperfection. Perfection is within, and causality and imperfection are without; even with bad genes, there is a prior embryonic recognition of a pattern of perfection. Even with chromosomal disorders, conventional doctors do not believe there is much we can do to alter the expression of those genes. Yet even patients with chromosomal disorders can be structurally supported with osteopathic treatment, such that they express as much of the plan of perfection as possible despite their genetic restrictions.

A good example of how osteopathic treatment can benefit even a patient with a genetic disorder is Down syndrome. Down syndrome is a disorder resulting from an extra, third copy of chromosome number 13. A hallmark of this disorder is mental retardation and specific facial characteristics (including a large tongue, small eyes, flattened nasal bridge, and smaller head and body size). Early on in my path to relearning traditional osteopathy, I saw multiple cases of children with genetic diseases whose development was improved compared to kids who did not receive osteopathic treatment. The typical flattened nasal bridge was not so flattened in treated children, for instance. Rather, the nasal bridges and total facial appearance in these treated children were so normal that without pretreatment photos I would not have believed they had a genetic abnormality. In terms of outward appearances, they would not be identified as having Down syndrome.

Another dramatic example of the supportive nature of traditional osteopathic treatment on genetic disorders occurred later in my educational journey. At an advanced traditional osteopathy conference, I observed a child with a rare chromosomal disorder (called a 9p deletion disorder). He was 9 years old and had just learned to walk after receiving multiple osteopathic treatments over the years. There is only one other child in the United States with this rare genetic disorder. The other child's doctor, an M.D., was present at the conference and remarked at how much better this child was doing. He even entertained the idea of sending his patient to California for traditional osteopathic treatment.

An example from my personal practice, an older mother brought her 3-year-old Down syndrome child in for evaluation. He was small for his age: his height, weight, and head circumference were more in line with the measurements one would see for a one-year-old. He had speech delay, and a lopsided cone head for which he wore a helmet for several months. The conventional pediatricians and specialists she had consulted said there was nothing that could be done, because this was all part of his genetic picture. The child's mother, however, felt that there was something more than just the genetic disorder manifesting.

Several days after the first osteopathic treatment, both parents noticed that he was speaking more. I believe the plagiocephaly helmet had restricted his head growth and his development. I do *not* believe that my one osteopathic treatment allowed his plan of perfection to manifest, despite his genetic defect. Rather, I believe that I got these immediate results because I specifically and precisely reduced the compression forces of the helmet. On their return, I asked more questions to see if there were other mechanical constraints upon his development, such as any other traumas. The mother became offended when I asked the details of how and why she massaged him daily. Down syndrome children have low muscle tone from head to toe, and it is generally not advisable to massage anyone with low muscle tone. A conventional outside observer would say that this one treatment improved his speech despite his genetics. In this case, I never got the chance to fully investigate his plan of perfection overlaid by a genetic disorder.

I look at all of my patients and I see derailment from the plan of perfection. The events that happen in our lives to alter our tensions, our choices to allow procedures to be done upon us. . . every action has a consequence. When the consequences, the strains, pile up and our physical bodies can no longer bear it, we suffer.

MORE PHILOSOPHY

Very few of us escape this life without some degree of physical trauma. How much trauma, and to what degree, can determine the path we end up on and how much we suffer.

For the longest time, I believed my T-bone car accident was the primary derailment of my life, and that it was the main cause of my physical suffering. Ten years later, I understand that an intubation, four wisdom teeth extractions and two pregnancies also contributed to the exacerbation of my pain. Recently, after several months of self-treatment, I have further concluded that two earlier traumatic injuries in my childhood derailed me from perfect health. At 7 years old, I stuck a wire coat hanger into an electrical outlet. It sparked and scared me so badly that I dropped it. I don't know why I was not injured at the time. But I am now convinced that I became altered, that this event was my *primary* derailment. All that I was and all that I became as I grew and developed into adulthood (including symptoms of ADHD) can now be explained.

I am no longer hyperactive. Skeptics would say that age has slowed me down, and while that may true, most ADHD or ADD patients will tell you that the mind also races. My brain is now calm. It no longer races. Because it is now calm, I can look back at what it used to be, and see that it was not good. How and why my electrocution or electrical shock caused my hyperactivity issues is a subject for another book, one on the electrical philosophy of osteopathy. For now, the other major injury in my childhood, which I have come to consider as a tertiary derailment from perfect health, was a blunt force facial trauma (the car accident is now bumped down to a secondary derailment). When I was about 8 years old, I took a lemon to the face, dead center between the eyes. I believe that that impact contributed to my later allergies in adulthood (this will be explained later in the segment on allergies in Chapter 4). The fact that I no longer suffer from these allergies, which allows me to reflect back how I achieved my results, also grants me hindsight as to causation. The fact that I get similar results from my patients leads me to broader conclusions as to how the physical body suffers. Many of my patients, as we clear up their problems, come to see and even list the major derailment events that led them to their current state of physical suffering. Treating all pertinent vectors at once at major body areas allows for precision, efficiency and instantaneous tissue changes at the areas of contact.

How *long* the physical body suffers is another matter altogether. It is up to the patient to seek answers. If they are satisfied with conventional pills because they are quick and provide temporary results, most patients will stay with the conventional approach. The smaller percentage of the population demands answers and explanations. Many of my patients, who are new to traditional osteopathy, invariably ask, "Why haven't I heard of this before?" If they get results and the suffering of their physical body decreases, or even ends, they always get to this question. Every patient gets the explanations from Chapter 1; hence this book, which I hope reaches all of you who still suffer and want to make *sense* of your or your child's suffering.

How do I understand my patients' suffering? Because this lost art is so difficult to explain to the uninitiated, the skills required in order to achieve instantaneous results come at a great financial and personal cost, and because there are so few of us traditional osteopathic physicians, I find it remarkable that people find me at all. We are hidden and will continue to be hidden. Patients who find me accidentally or by word of mouth early within the first year of their suffering, I deem very fortunate. Those who find traditional osteopathy late, and who suffer for years before finally getting results, I conclude that they *had* to suffer. They had to learn to ask questions and seek. They would have to become disenchanted with conventional medicine, if not completely distrustful of it. They would have to be open to looking at other options. Then, they would have to have (or else learn to have) an awareness of how those other options affect their body. They would have to use their common sense to distinguish by trial and error if this option is the correct path. It becomes a journey where patience has to be learned. There is also a component of faith needed to continue the seeking; otherwise, they stop searching. The lesson is that suffering is *necessary* so that we can learn and eventually be better for it.

FIGURE 1:

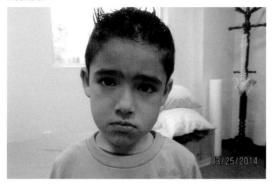

This photo was taken after JV came in, complaining of a headache several weeks after a car accident. Note the tilt of his head, caused by spasms on the left side of his neck.

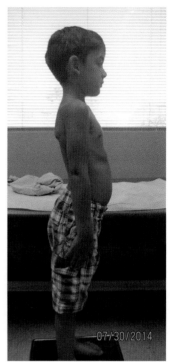

Note the upswing of JV's back side and the protuberant abdomen.

FIGURE 2:

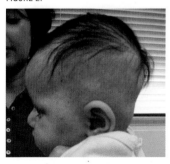

SU was a screaming, fussy infant who would often cry for three hours a day. Note the knobby and bulbous parts of her head.

FIGURE 3:

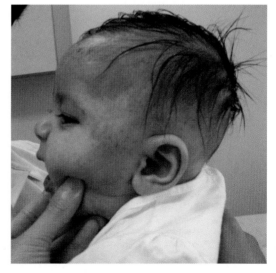

One week later her head is more rounded and she is less fussy.

FIGURE 4:

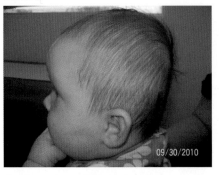 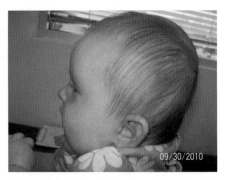

Note the roundness at the forehead and the flatness at the back of the head.

After treatment, the forehead is not so prominent and the back of the head has rounded out.

FIGURE 5:

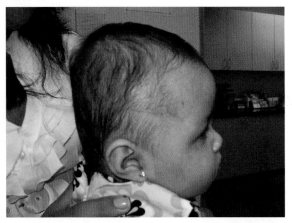

Note that DB's cone head was shaped by being wedged down low in the birth canal, while her twin brother sat breech on top of her in the womb.

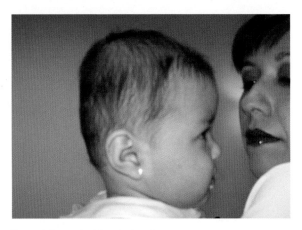

She needed approximately 25 treatments.

FIGURE 6:

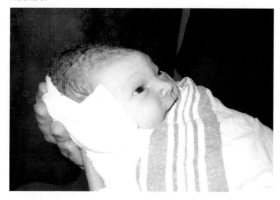

CB's head was stuck in the birth canal, and he was pulled out with a vacuum. Note the large red welt left by the vacuum.

FIGURE 7:

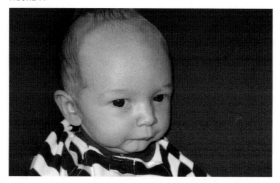

This is CB at 7 weeks of age. Note the prominent ridging of the bones in the middle of his forehead and by the left ear, crossing over his head onto the other side. Also important is the placement of his lower jaw: it is pulled back. This is not a coincidence; imagine the future orthodontic work he will need to align his jaw and teeth.

FIGURE 8:

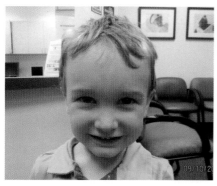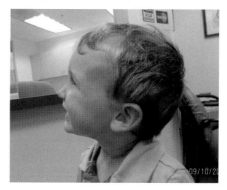

This is CB 3 years later. Note the near perfect symmetry of eyes, eyebrows, and cheeks.

Note the jawline. It is no longer pulled back.

FIGURE 9:

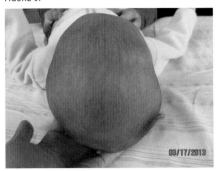

This is DOF at 3 months of age. The forehead is prominent on the left and sloping toward the right. The area behind the left ear is flattened, while the area near the right ear is bulbous and has a tuft of hair. Both are evidence that this area is not as compressed.

FIGURE 10:

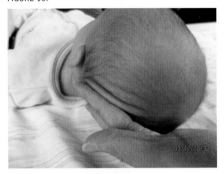

In the womb, the scalp is stretched and smoothed out by the bones. On this side, the extra skin folds demonstrate the underlying bones are still compressed from the birth process.

FIGURE 11:

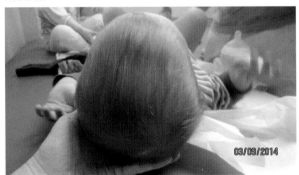

Note the symmetry one year later.

FIGURE 12:

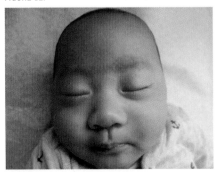

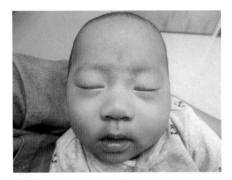

In this pretreatment photo, there doesn't seem to be anything significantly wrong with KL at first glance. He just looks like a small, premature baby.

After osteopathic treatment, we can now see that his forehead looks more rounded. The dome of his head is now proportional to his cheeks.

FIGURE 13:

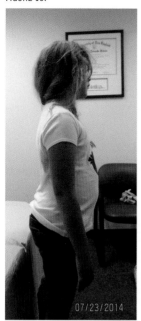

07/23/2014

Note the curved backside, with the buttocks being pulled high and tight. Also, the abdomen is quite protuberant.

FIGURE 14:

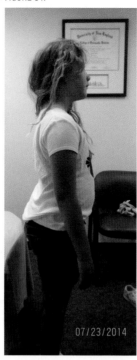

07/23/2014

After treatment, some balance has returned; the backside is more flattened, as is the abdomen.

FIGURE 15:

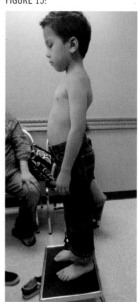

Here, JW has the same posture—the high and tight arched lower back. This tight posture does not allow him to disperse his weight load/tensions down through the leg. Rather, his weight load and tensions are borne directly onto the feet, causing them to roll in.

FIGURE 16:

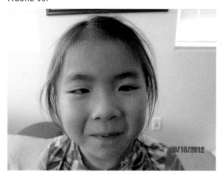

At first inspection, we only notice the most prominent feature of her face: her crossed eye.

FIGURE 17:

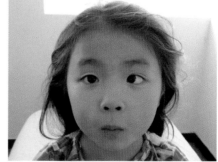

Forty minutes after this first treatment, we can see that not only have her eyes changed, but there are differences in her whole face.

FIGURE 18:

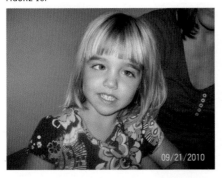

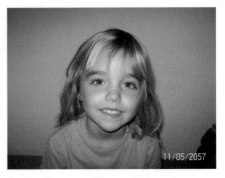

KN asked her mother to find someone to help her with her eye.

Four visits later, we are all happy with the results.

FIGURE 19:

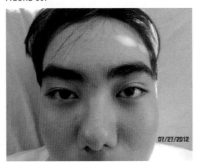

As a young child, NT had corrective surgery for esotropia. Years later, asymmetries in the face are evident.

FIGURE 20:

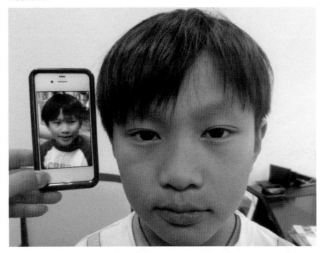

These two photos were taken one week apart.

FIGURE 21:

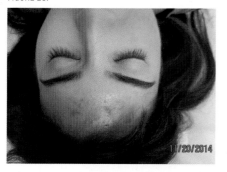 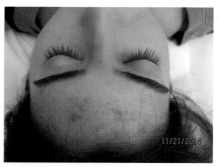

Before treatment, her skin is oily, her acne appears inflamed and the pustules appear ready to burst.

Thirty minutes after treatment, the acne pustules appear to be less red and angry.

FIGURE 22a:

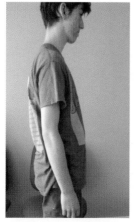 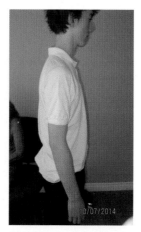

In this pre-treatment photo of SE, his head is pitched forward. He is mechanically inefficient. His postural muscles have to keep him upright and pull him back from tumbling forward.

After treatment, his head is more in line with his neck and back. This posture requires less work and he can be more relaxed.

FIGURE 22b:

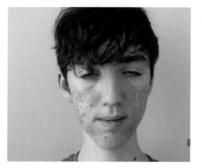 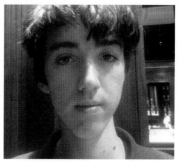

SE's acne is nodular, inflamed and painful.

SE is happy with his progress, and allowed his mom to take this photo.

FIGURE 23:

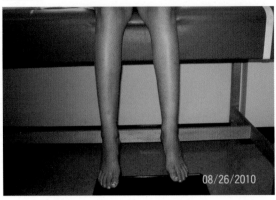

The outward angulation of the left lower leg is most likely caused by muscle spasms following the trauma that caused the broken ankle. As she grew, the muscles continue to be contracted. This chronic contracted state makes the leg appear and function as if it is shorter, which in turns causes her hips to be uneven while standing up.

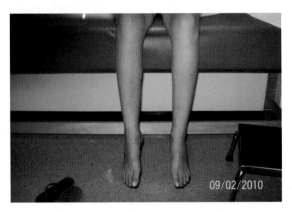

After the second treatment, KK's leg looks more normal. Her scoliosis has "disappeared."

FIGURE 24:

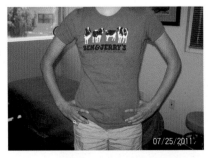

MM's whole right side appears smaller, tighter and more contracted.

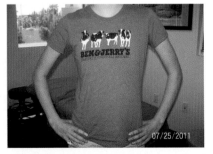

After treatment, the right hip appears more relaxed and dropped. The right side now looks a little more elongated.

PART III

MEDICAL PROBLEMS WITH STRUCTURAL CAUSES

PART III: OVERVIEW

Finding the precise cause of a patient's current issues requires hunting for the tissues or injuries responsible. Tracing backward in a patient's traumatic history is what allows us as osteopaths to find clues as to where we should be looking. Precision is key, not only to the efficacy of osteopathic treatment but also to avoid altering the vectors themselves, which can result in more harm than good. The conventional medical approach is so dramatically different from the traditional osteopathic approach. For the osteopath, once an affected area is treated, if there are results, then it proves both the cause and the effect. Conventionally, most doctors do not recognize the role that mechanical trauma plays in all aspects of our health—even our allergies can be traced back to past trauma! This insistence on seeking a biochemical cause where a mechanical cause is responsible, coupled with an over-reliance on pharmaceutical response, is what obligates patients to see the difference between allopathic and osteopathic care, and make the choice that is right for them.

CHAPTER 11

Infants
(Birth to 1 year)

W HEN THE conventional medical system (CMS) looks at a medical problem, it calls it a "disease" and seeks to alter the body's current state with powerful biochemistry, through the use of pharmaceuticals. If it is a chronic condition, modern medicine seeks to delay its progression or alter its course with chronic medications. Even preventing worsening symptoms seems to require chronic medication in the eyes of the conventional medical system. Structural diseases (those with a mechanical component) are addressed with surgery. For example, a lump or bump within a closed tissue area may press on vital structures and need to be removed. When I evaluate a patient, I like to ask myself, "What caused this patient to deviate from the normal state of health?" I ask about traumas all the way back into childhood. I will even go so far as to ask about birth history (as we saw in the previous chapter, there are any number of potential traumas that can occur during the fetal and post-birth period). In this chapter, I hope to provide clues and explanations so that parents and patients may come to the understanding that mechanical traumas at different stages of development can contribute to lasting "disease" later in life. And, just as importantly, I hope to show the ways in which these traumas can be healed.

The chronic problems that present in infants during their first year of life can be attributed to structural strains from the in-utero environment in the prenatal period, and especially the birth history. In the osteopathic evaluation of an infant, we ask about all the events leading up to the birth in detail. It is also very helpful to have video or photographs, as there are multiple vectors of strain that can be imparted upon the newborn's head and neck. In a vaginal delivery, as the fetal head "engages," the head is circumferentially compressed—the baby's head is tucked and the baby spirals out. As the head crowns, maternal contractions push on the baby; in the final push, the baby has to hyperextend the head, neck, and upper back. I find that for a normal first vaginal delivery, the babies that do well are the ones that deliver after 8–16 hours of labor. Any birth that is too fast may cause problems, because the bones of the skull will not slowly lock down symmetrically. This means that as the newborn head attempts to grow, unloading of the compression occurs asymmetrically, and the infant experiences twisting strain in the skull base. For labors that go on far beyond the 16-hour mark, the bones and tissues are so compressed that the infant cannot naturally decompress on its own. The mechanically compressed infant skull will present in different ways; early in infancy, nursing (and the work associated with it) uses the muscles of the mouth, jaw, face, and neck, freeing them up and decompressing mild cranial strains resulting from an uncomplicated birth. Through normal growth, the outward growth and stretch of tissues is sometimes enough to continue the decompression of the compressed infant skull.

COLIC: THE FUSSY SCREAMING INFANT

It is estimated that 1 in 5 infants will have colic, a ratio which translates to about 700,000 babies per year in the United States alone.[21] The usual pattern that plays out in colic cases is blood-curdling screams from the baby, which cause the family to rush the infant to the ER, only to be turned away with a diagnosis of "colic." They receive reassurances that there is nothing dangerous or life-threatening affecting their child. But a diagnosis is not an explanation, and the parents have not been given what they seek: an explanation and a cure.

Conventionally, parents are told to do nothing—that the infant will outgrow this period. In fact, they do *not* outgrow the problem of compressive loading on the skull. I believe that they only adapt to the tensions, that is, they learn to live with it. The screaming infant is feeling tension from head to toe as its body tries to expand and elongate its form. If there is resistance from the vectors of birth strain that the baby cannot match or even circumferentially push out against, there will be tension—which can manifest as pain. The louder the scream, the more the severe is the headache. I have long suspected that they are suffering from migraine pain (and several researchers agree).[22, 23, 24]

In physically examining an infant, there are signs that a parent may find that will explain the fussiness.

I teach parents to look at their infant for the following:

- Soft spot

- Green, bulging scalp veins

- Red, splotchy red skin on the face, forehead, and scalp

- Flatness of the back or one side of the head

The soft spot is an area where the bones of the skull should not yet meet. Babies whose heads are still too compressed will have a small, tight soft spot. Often the spot will be "poofy"; when the baby is laid on its back, the soft spot gets "poofier." This change that occurs with a change in position is an indication of increasing head pressure. The infant will start to fuss and wants to be picked up so that gravity drains some blood. These fussy periods can vary, ranging from one hour to five hours. Theoretically, babies treated by an osteopathic physician should manifest changes immediately, if the unloading of the compression is precisely reduced. I educate my patient's parents on these findings and the expected changes. The soft spot should soften and widen, and appear more like a pothole. Bulging green scalp veins will bulge less, and the beet red skin of suffused blood and vascular congestion should clear up immediately. A good treatment results in a pulsating soft spot, which is reflective of the heart action pumping blood into the skull. That there is now pulsation implies that venous outflow is unimpeded, allowing for a net movement of flow and pressures coming in *and* going out. This should coincide with a mellow and happier baby. A profound treatment that results in instantaneous appearance of the soft spot pulsation is difficult to achieve, and very few osteopathic physicians can do this. As a result, my patient's parents typically do not note the pulsation until after several visits.

SU is a colicky baby, who would fuss and scream for three hours a day. Before our treatment, her head shape was odd, with the forehead being bulbous (see Figure 2 in the photo insert). The front of her head was also very sloped, while the back area behind and just above the left ear were very compressed. You can see that she has little to no hair in this area; this represents poor blood exchange and flow. Her head appeared to be stuck and painfully tight. One week later (as seen in Figure 3 in the photo insert), the shape of her head seems more normal. Hair has started to fill in the sparse area. She is much happier, although she needed several more visits.

I have witnessed a profound treatment of colic, when my mentor Dr. Herb Miller, treated my 3-month-old baby. The back of her head was starting to flatten out, her head was starting to twist, and we had been having problems nursing. In twenty minutes, he gave her back to me. Her blue veins had disappeared and the soft spot had started pulsating. That night was the first time in her life that we nursed in bed and fell asleep together. It was a beautiful moment. As she has grown up, her eyes, mouth, and lips are nearly perfectly symmetrical. Her hips and legs are near perfect in symmetry of motion. By my estimation, at the peak of his knowledge, wisdom, and experience in retirement, that one treatment lasted her 18 months.

One research article from Korea found that colic "can lead to disorders of behavioral and emotional regulation at the toddler stage such as sleep and feeding disorders, chronic fussiness, excessive clinginess, and temper tantrums".[25] Another article found that there are structural brain changes in the adult, attributable to their temperament as 4-month-old infants.[26] Still other studies are trying to strategize methods to treat colic.[27, 28, 29, 30, 31, 32] Below is a chart adapted from the Korean study, where developmental, age-related issues are typical. I commonly see and treat these types of behaviors; is it possible that they are directly related?

Age (in years)	0	1	2	3	4	5	6	7
Excessive Crying	X	X	X					
Head-Banging	X	X	X					
Feeding/Nursing Problems		X	X	X	X			
Nocturnal Waking			X	X	X			
Temper Tantrums			X	X	X			
Biting/Hitting/Scratching				X	X	X	X	X
Night Terrors					X	X	X	
Hyperactivity						X	X	X
Enuresis							X	X

LATCHING AND NURSING ISSUES

We have seen that babies can sometimes be found sucking their thumbs in the womb. We do know that the reflex to suck and swallow is present in the fetus at 32 weeks of gestation; premature infants born before 32 weeks need to stay in a NICU and learn to suck and swallow before they can be released from the hospital. We also know that planned, C-sectioned babies in fairly uncomplicated pregnancies generally do not have problems with latching and nursing. In vaginally delivered infants with latching and nursing issues, the question becomes one of determining the factor that has altered and affected their ability to nurse. I would suggest that the pressures, compressive loads, twist, and shears in the birth process have altered the tensions in the newborn's head, face, neck and mouth, so that something as natural as feeding is now difficult. I would say that the baby does not latch or nurse well because *it can't*.

Nursing requires a complex coordination of the muscles of the mouth, tongue, and throat. Parents can evaluate their child's efforts to nurse by letting the baby suck on a middle finger (turned upward, so that the nail is in direct contact with the baby's tongue). The normal, healthy infant should open wide enough to get the finger/nipple in. The tongue should push up against the finger/nipple/pacifier and pull it back into the back of the mouth and throat. The movement of the tongue should create a vacuum effect and draw the finger back further as the baby swallows. With normal nursing, you should see the muscles of the mouth, jaw, and neck move in a coordinated manner. All this can be observed from the side, just in front of, around, behind, and beneath the infant's temporomandibular joint (TMJ).

Babies have different tensions, depending on which stage of latching and nursing they have difficulty with. Babies that cannot open their mouth wide enough to latch onto the breast are caught in an upward shear and hyperextension. Babies that just clamp down and gum the breast are compressed all around the skull and jammed down into the neck. Babies that cannot coordinate the vacuum sucking and swallowing are caught in the phase of posterior head compression, where two cranial nerves that supply the back of the tongue and throat are compressed.

In treating the infant, I have the mother attempt breastfeeding. While I treat the head, the mother can feel the instantaneous change in the latch, suck, and swallow. In theory, the molding forces of a vaginal birth compound slowly over time, allowing for passage of the newborn cranium. As the days progress and as the newborn head continues to stretch out the compression, unfold, and unmold, the first treatment's effects dissipate. I ask the parents to observe how long a treatment lasts; usually, the more difficult the labor, the more compression load the infant skull must bear, and the shorter the effects of a first treatment. With each successive treatment (as the infant cranium unmolds) the results last longer and the visits are spaced farther apart.

PLAGIOCEPHALY AND TORTICOLLIS

Since 1992, when the American Academy of Pediatrics first made the recommendations for infant sleep positioning on the back or side, physicians have noticed a dramatic increase in plagiocephaly, an abnormal shape of the head.[33] One side of the head is flattened, while the other side may be normal and round. The face and eyes may appear uneven or perhaps appear lopsided (parents often describe the shape as "cone-headed"). The abnormal head shape may be accompanied by a neck muscle spasm (called the sternocleidomastoid muscle) causing the head to turn and tilt, restricting the motion of the head on the neck.

One major medical center reported a six-fold increase in the cases of plagiocephaly.[34] The most conservative treatment approach for plagiocephaly is alternating and changing the infant's head position. Seventy-three percent of infants with simple positional plagiocephaly resolve their cranial and facial asymmetry by an average follow-up age of 10.5 months.[35] Yet that still leaves a large percentage requiring further intervention, whether it is helmet therapy (a counterintuitive and even controversial option) or even surgery. Helmet therapy is the application of a measured and molded helmet to restrict growth on the area that is most lopsided. Most parents report that the infant grabs at the helmet, indicating that the child is uncomfortable. I object to helmet therapy; as a pediatrician who conducts regular well-child checks, I measure the circumference of the head to plot growth over time. Ideally, growth should be outward in all directions, like a balloon. The molding helmet puts a compressive vector at a bony prominence (where there is too much growth). It does nothing to encourage growth in the restricted area. Osteopathic work seeks to unload and reduce compression vectors; why would we approve a technology that *causes* more compression?

The problem is primarily one of compression. A precise treatment should be *de-compression*. Furthermore, our understanding of the compression is that it occurs at the cranial base, which then leads to the more obvious asymmetries in the face and crown. Helmet therapy attempts to correct the outward appearance in the upper portion of the crown (or cranial vault). And yet, in a long-term study (well after helmet therapy was completed) it was found that both the cranial base and the cranial vault measurements had regressed.[36] The asymmetry is a symptom, an effect of a cranial base compression. Traditional cranial osteopathy addresses the cause and not the effect, that is, the "disease." To make matters worse, helmet therapy is not without its complications, including pressure sores, discomfort for the infant, and failure to correct the deformity.[36]

Another study evaluated teenagers between 12 and 17 years of age. The incidence of plagiocephaly was found to be only 1.1 percent.[37] As the child grows up, most cases of plagiocephaly, therefore, seem to resolve on their own, and some suggest that infants are being over-treated. The question to consider thus becomes: is there harm in under-treatment? Several studies have associated plagiocephaly with neurodevelopmental issues, learning issues for language, speech, and academic performance, chronic ear infections, and dental bite issues.[38, 39, 40, 41, 42]

While most plagiocephaly occurs alone, torticollis can be associated with it. Torticollis is a spasm in a muscle called the stenocleidomastoid (located on either side of the neck) that causes the head to bend on one side while tilting on the opposite side. The answer as to which was the initial cause is still unknown. The incidence of torticollis in the newborn population is only 16 percent.[43] There has also been a reported association of "stuck" positioning and labor and delivery issues, which would support the osteopathic concept that mechanical compressive prenatal and perinatal loading causes problems in newborns.

Lopsided heads and twisting at the neck are intertwined in the birth process, and result from the complex overlay of multiple vectors of a normal birth process. Add minor pregnancy complications and false contractions, or include a prolonged labor over 18 hours or one that ultimately ends up in a C-section; all difficulties and complications will factor into the severity of the lopsidedness. The important goal is to free up enough tensions so that the baby can have freedom and symmetric range of motion in the head and neck. The severity will influence how much time and how many visits it takes to balance out. Most parents tell me that they see their child turning more freely on the same day. Often, we see the head shape begin to round out during the first visit.

The conventional approach when the infant head is mildly misshapen is conservative: the "wait and see" approach. The following cases highlight the varying degrees of difficulty of treating a lopsided head. Treatment length and time depend on multiple variables in the prenatal and perinatal environment. Traditional osteopathic treatments for these infants are primarily cranial osteopathy because the strain patterns are primarily compressive forces acquired at the time of birth. Unique to any other philosophy of medicine, only traditional cranial osteopathy *decompresses*. There have been studies done in the US,[44] Canada[45] and Italy[46] using cranial osteopathy for the treatment of plagiocephaly that show benefit. Below, these treatment photos will also demonstrate results.

KL is a happy baby with no real medical issues. Her mother was concerned about the flattening of the back of her head. During the birth process, as the baby drops down in the birth canal, the chin is tucked down. The whole head is then compressed, mostly from front to back. You can see in the photos in Figure 4 (see the photo insert) that, as she developed in the first several months of life, the back area did not free up enough and decompress. Because her back was not rounding out, growth in the front was not as restricted; as a result, the forehead is rather prominent. The area behind the left ear at the *bottom* of the skull (where she is restricted) is the *cause* of her issues. A helmet, which would place a restrictive band around the *top* of the head, is essentially a Band-Aid® for the symptoms of the lopsided head. She responded immediately and dramatically to one osteopathic treatment. The flattened area behind her ear is much improved. Although it is not perfect, she now has enough freedom that in time this area will be able to grow and balance.

DB is a twin who was predominantly head-down in utero, while her brother sat on top of her in a breech position. She was molded in this environment for quite a while. Her mother was concerned about the flatness at the back of her head (see Figure 5 in the photo insert). She did not want her to have helmet therapy. DB required about 25 visits. This was a difficult case because the molding occurred even before the cartilage in her skull became bone. We had to wait for her to grow in order to take advantage of some of the natural decompression that goes along with growth.

CB's mother was worried by the way his face, head, and jaw were growing. He was born vaginally, but required help from vacuum suction to pull him out (see Figure 6 in the photo insert). Note the welt left by the vacuum on his head. In Figure 7 (in the photo insert), taken several weeks later, the posterior shear of the vacuum was still pulling the soft tissue of his face tight across the underlying bony structure. His face and jaw were still stuck in the pattern of a posterior shearing injury. He only needed about seven treatments from 5 months to 10 months. The final two photos, in Figure 8 in the photo insert, are from a 3-year follow-up. He gets a lot of compliments. Most of his head shape is due to the difficult birth. Yet a good cranial osteopathic treatment does all things at once, unloading the traumatic forces and decompressing.

DOF is a happy baby, with a pleasant personality. The only problem was that his mom was increasingly distressed at his flattened and lopsided head. She refused the helmet, and asked if I could help him.

On inspection, the flattened left side of his head was demonstrated to have extra folds of scalp (see Figure 9 in the photo insert). I inferred that the three cranial bones on this side behind the left ear (temporal, parietal, and occiput) are jammed (see Figure 10 in the photo insert). In infants, growth of the head comes from growth of the skull. The skull is formed from pieces which are pushed outward by the growing brain. C-sectioned babies rarely have extra folds of scalp. During the birth process, this area in the back of the head was compressed. It was a long, rough delivery and he did not decompress sufficiently. On the right side, there is a prominent bony bulge. Just behind that on the scalp, he has a long tuft of hair. From these top-down views, his head shape almost looks like a parallelogram. Helmet therapy would put a band-like compression at the bottom right (where the tuft of hair is located) to slow the knobby, bulbous growth of *brain* and bone. These physical findings have a mechanical basis. The cause is not genetic, and the physical signs are not coincidental. In Figure 11 in the photo insert (taken one year later) you can see the dramatic effects that treatment had on improving the symmetry of his head shape.

REFLUX/SPIT UPS

Thirty percent of newborns have reflux, and most newborns will have some degree of spit ups. From small to large spit ups, the volume reflects the degree of compression of the newborn head. Conventional approaches to reflux used to be the administration of anti-reflux medications, which now have fallen out of favor because of long-term cardiac side effect risks. In place of medications, the new conservative approach is an older approach of observation and reflux precautions of small, frequent feeds, frequent burping while feeding, and upright positioning after feeding. For severe cases, the last resort would be surgery. The osteopathic, mechanical approach involves compression of the delicate area in back of the head and at the base of the skull. Three cranial nerves—the ninth cranial nerve (CN IX), the twelfth cranial nerve (CN XII) and the tenth cranial nerve (CN X)—are responsible for the tongue and vegetative functions, respectively. The ninth and the tenth exit out at the back of the head, while the twelfth exits through its very own little tunnel at the back of the head. All three may be kinked and compressed through a difficult labor.

Reflux is an uncomfortable problem. The tissue in the esophagus is burned by the acid, as it is not designed for it—its sole purpose is for forward transport of food. All reflux babies arch. Most people, even including general pediatricians, believe that they arch to extend the head and neck, partly because of the gas and partly because of the pain that accompanies an episode of reflux. Most people marvel at the strength of the refluxing newborn neck and its ability to hold up the head so soon. My osteopathic understanding of this arching is that it is not the infant's reaction to acid at all. My colleagues and I believe it to be a problem of the tightness of the muscles of head, neck, and back, where the tensions from birth are still present. Tightness and compression at the base of the skull and neck explains the full gamut of behaviors. The cranial nerves exiting through openings in the skull base are crimped from the birth compression, while at the same time the resting length of the tissues, the pre-muscles, are shorter (because they are more compressed) and allow for mechanical advantage, requiring less work to lift up the head.

For example: KL was born premature at 32 weeks. His mom brought him in because he had spit ups of varying volume. As he aged, his mother noticed that on days of large volume spit ups, he would be fussier and arch his head and neck more. She would take him to me for treatment, he would get better, and then he would try to grow. He would come up against the resistance of his prior preemie compression history and the soft spot would tighten. He would arch, get fussy, and spit up more. He would continue this pattern of spitting up, improving after treatment, growing, and spitting up again through his first year of life. His mom could tell just from his behavior when he needed to come in. With infants, we like to take advantage of their continued growth and treat them as they try to expand. Before treatment, his head looked a little narrowed and pointy (see the first photo in Figure 12 in the photo insert). After treatment, it is a larger, rounder skull that is more proportional to his cheeks (see the second photo in Figure 12 in the photo insert).

The issue with prematurity is not so much the size of the cranium; rather, it is an issue of it being composed of more water than tissue. In the passage of a round cranial structure, whose size is as small as a navel orange and whose consistency resembles flan, we see more compressive strain than compared to a baby at full term, whose head is the size of a small grapefruit with the consistency of Jell-O. Not only does the preemie head have to deal with forces during the birth process for which it is not properly developed, but once delivered the infant body now also has to deal with the repetitive stress of gravitational forces upon the brain cells.

CHRONIC CONGESTION

Every now and then I come across an infant where the parents report his having congestion "from the day he was born." In normal deliveries, where the face is down and the back of the head crowns (called *occiput anterior*) the face and nose can be compressed in the earliest stage of birth. As the head drops down into the birth canal, the chin is tucked and the head is squeezed down front to back or back to front. At birth, decompression did not happen and the face and nose continue to be "stuck." The more common mechanical cause of chronic congestion is the face presentation, or the infant being born "sunny side up." These babies will have more problems because the early facial bones and tissues ride under the maternal bony pubic symphysis. Their face is effectively "squeegeed" against hard bone. It is very difficult for the infant to decompress on its own from that type of bony pressure. Occasionally, breastfeeding and growth of the face and head allow for decompression of the upper nasal passages in the normal facedown position. Often, the faceup position cannot decompress on its own, even with breastfeeding, growth, and the passage of time. When the face is compressed front to back, with a combined downward drag, these infants will have nursing issues. This can be readily assessed by checking the sucking and swallowing the infant does on one's finger.

CHRONIC EAR INFECTIONS

Chronic ear infections represent one of the most common mechanical issues in pediatrics. Chronic ear infections are caused by a lack of drainage, where pooling of secretions or formula (from bottle feeding or even breastfeeding at night) in the middle ear causes infection. Most conventional family doctors and pediatricians are not taught that the bones in the head move, or that these subtle motions allow for respiration and ventilation of the sinuses and ears. The idea that this results in airflow in the respiratory tract and drainage of fluid in the middle ear is difficult for most physicians to believe, as it is so contrary to what they are conventionally taught. Chronic ear infections are always treated, at first, with multiple rounds of antibiotics. Sometimes for older children allergy medications and decongestants are medical options. Persistent chronic ear infections that increase the risk of permanent hearing loss are always surgically treated. The question is, why isn't the fluid draining the natural way, by way of the Eustachian tube? Why must we cut a hole in the eardrum, the tympanic membrane? The membrane needs to be intact for the transmission of sounds for hearing. The surgical fix is itself just a quick fix, one that does not answer the question of "why?"

The conventional approach would be the placement of ear tubes, a surgical procedure performed by an ENT (ear, nose, and throat) specialist to drain and ventilate the middle ear. Cranial osteopathic treatment frees up the cranial bones and allows them to move and drain the middle ears naturally. Dr. Andrew Weil recommends cranial osteopathy and has just concluded a National Institute of Health study at the University of Arizona looking at using cranial osteopathy and echinacea for the treatment of chronic ear infections.[47]

CHAPTER 12

Toddlers (1–2 years) and Children (2–10 years)

A FTER THE first year of life and once they've learned to walk, children get a little more freedom and independence. Some personalities will take to this newfound freedom quickly, while others will be more cautious. Watching children take these steps can offer osteopathic physicians insight as to where tensions are arising in the body. Often, children will cause themselves acute injury by falling. When observing their movements, it is also important to note how they transition from standing to sitting, and how they climb off a chair. A single activity or behavior, repeated often enough, can induce a repetitive stress in their body.

Falls are always harmful, though they can be deceptively so. A little fall sometimes is not enough to elicit caution from parents. But from my experience, trauma always begets more traumas, in a vicious circle, whether there is head trauma or not.

BEHAVIOR

I often instruct parents to observe changes in their children's behavior as being signs of their not feeling good. Children can be quick to snap; they do not have the words or understanding that something has disrupted them from their usual pattern of normal. Removed from normal and wound up with tensions, they cannot sleep and cannot rest. This can be observed most readily in boys; in the 1–2 year age range, they may throw toys, be more clingy and fussy, and hit others. Little girls can also be fussy or clingy when they don't feel well, although they tend not to be as destructive. In the week following an osteopathic treatment, parents report their child being calmer and easier to manage and more direct. I believe that this delay in the change in behavior is attributable to better sleep.

Sleep

Behavior can also be linked to sleep, lack of sleep, or poor quality of sleep. Parents can readily assess this relationship. They know if their child is "hard to put down." In medical terminology, we say that the patient has difficulty in sleep initiation. Children who wake up frequently do not reach the deep stages of sleep, and are easy to rouse. These are children with issues of sleep maintenance. Waking up early may not be a sleep disorder, so long as the child wakes up happy and alert. The quality of the sleep can be deduced by observing how the child is positioned through the night. If there is a lot of shifting and movement, these are called sleep disorders, same as they are in the adult population. Tossing and turning is just as indicative of restless sleep in children as it is in adults.

There are multiple safe strategies available to help parents cycle or sleep train their child. One safe strategy for infancy and toddlerhood is the pacifier. Up until the formation of the teeth, I generally feel that pacifiers do have their place. In the normal state, without a pacifier, the tongue molds and shapes the roof of the mouth. The palate forms from three early bony pieces that come together and fuse to form the outer hard palate. Deeper in the mouth, the bony edge of the hard palate has a fleshier part called the soft palate. If the infant needs and wants a pacifier, I generally advise finding a broader one that is soft and pliable. Often the hospital pacifiers are too hard and narrow.

In terms of the structural tensions in the body, from head to toe, contributing to poor sleep, an osteopathic treatment can usually show its direct relationship as immediately as during the treatment itself. I find that when precisely reducing the patient's vectors, the effects carry over through to several days.

SWAYBACK OR EXCESSIVE LUMBAR LORDOSIS

During their early structural period, all toddlers have some degree of a mild curve or arch in their lower back. This low back curve may appear partially exaggerated because of padding from a diaper. In older children and adults, excessive lordosis will have a corresponding protuberant belly. The term "swayback" was used to describe this excessive curve in the low back. Today, the medical term is "lumbar lordosis." The tightness and tension will also pull the sacrum (the bone in between the two hip bones) high and also raise the buttocks high. Exaggerations in the lordosis are caused by tensions in the connective tissue areas between the lumbar spine and the sacrum. In an attempt to grow and elongate the trunk, the connective tissue cannot stretch due to trauma. If the connective tissue tensions in the back are tight, there are areas of the body where compensations can be made. Posture and gait will be affected; when the low back is tight, the hamstrings tend to be tight; when the hamstrings are tight, the calves are tight; when the calves are tight, the Achilles tendons are tight; and when the Achilles tendons are tight, the arches are affected.

If the tightness in the low back continues throughout the pelvis, the hips cannot swing to dissipate the force of the truncal weight load. The full gravitational force of an upright posture is borne down through to the feet, and the load is more than what the arch can support. In these cases, the arches will fall and the patient will have functional flat feet. A functional flattened arch is one that cannot perform the work of supporting weight. These feet, when at rest and not standing, will show a nice medial arch. This is a clue that the cause of the problem is not local in the feet, and that we must look upward.

If the tightness in the lower back, continuing downward into the back of the legs is evenly distributed, we will observe a high and tight arch. Young children can often be found to toe walk; some will bounce or spring their step onto the balls and toes of the feet. General pediatricians describe this as a "habitual" toe walk as opposed to a "pathological" toe walk. Pathology would require specialist referral, and may lead to a surgical recommendation.

The relationship of the tight low backside to the tensions in the lower leg is not taught in general pediatric orthopedic training. I came to understand this relationship many years after I completed my training, and after many years working with infants and children osteopathically. It is not immediately intuitive that these discrete muscle groups with differing functions should have any direct and dynamic relationship in sharing strain and distributing workload. It takes many years in the field to be able to palpate those connections, which have their basis in anatomy and embryology. These separate muscle groups are all connected through the fascial envelopes encasing them and connecting them to each other (in much the same way as the casing around sausage links) and to the bony skeletal framework (which has its own connective tissue casing).

If we look further upward above the low back, what can we expect to find? Are there other physical clues in the structure that will help guide us? Where can we look?

- Rib cage: Lower ribs flare out (which gives the appearance of a sunken chest) and the uppers ribs are flared down.

- Collarbone: Clavicles tend to grow uniformly; they should be straight to maximize the space between the neck and shoulders. The more scalloped clavicles are toward the center; the size of that space reflects the stage in life that an injury occurred—the smaller the space, the earlier it occurred.

- Shoulders: Often the shoulders appear rolled forward, small and narrowed; usually, this is caused by the same injury that caused the collarbone to scallop.

- Facial Asymmetry: Usually reflects strains early in infancy.

MH is a patient who I first treated in my general pediatric practice. She had been generally healthy when she stopped visiting me due to insurance issues. I had not seen her for several years until her parents brought her in for poor sleep and behavioral issues, which were leading to troubles in school. On initial inspection, her posture appeared abnormal: her low back arch (lordosis) appeared exaggerated and her belly appeared rather large (see Figure 13 in the photo insert). The most significant event in her recent medical history was a surgery for the removal of the tonsils and adenoids. I focused her treatment on undoing or reducing the superior shear from the intubation. The areas I treated were the head, neck, shoulders, sternum, ribs, and left hip. In the after treatment photo, we can see that her belly is less protuberant and the back arch is not as severe (see Figure 14 in the photo insert). It will take several more visits to reset the resting tensions in the tissues in her back. I gave her exercises and stretches to help flatten out the arch and drop the buttocks. These exercises to correct the intubation will need to be practiced for the rest of her lifetime, and are included in the last section of this book. The correction should make her trunk more cylindrical, the line of her body straighter, and distribute her weight down through her hips and legs more efficiently.

Abnormal Gait

In observing the way a child walks, most parents notice when there is asymmetry of one leg. Causes of abnormal gait may derive from tensions in the hip, knee or ankle and vary in the presentation. Children may limp; have one foot turn in or out; there can even be such asymmetry as to cause imbalance, leading to tripping and falling. The child may have a tendency to occasionally toe walk. Intermittent toe walking is reassuring, as it is a sign that the issue is less likely a neurologic problem. Rather, it reflects muscular tightness and tension: the child has an awareness of it and is making a subconscious effort to reduce that tension. Often, children feel discomfort when fully planting the heel, causing a stretch of the Achilles tendon. They reflexively relax that tension by pointing the toe downward. Sometimes, we see children bounce back and forth between toe walking and normal gait with planting of the heel. They seem to almost vacillate in between a state of tension and non-tension in the feet. Soon, this becomes a habit.

At the toddler stage, after several months of walking, when abnormal gait is observed, the cause can almost always be attributed to muscular and ligament tensions along the back. Increased tensions come about as the toddler tries to grow and elongate the trunk. Difficulties arrive early if the child experienced a long difficult birth, or worse, had a fall in early infancy or childhood.

JW is a good example. At a physical exam, his mother describes the patient as walking abnormally. When he steps, his ankles roll in. This type of walk is also described as ankle pronation. His arches fall and cave in with weight bearing. When he is seated, I could observe the appearance of a small arch (see Figure 15 in the photo insert). So, we would say that his feet are normal in their structure because it has the form of an anatomic arch. There is simply something different about him when he stands and walks. Conventionally, orthopedists and physical therapists will look at this as a local problem and diagnose the cause as being loose or weak ligaments in his feet and ankles. The treatment would then be to put in arch supports and continue to resize and refit as his feet grow. The osteopathic approach looks at this problem of ankle pronation as one of weight bearing, postural, muscular, and ligamentous tension imbalance throughout the body.

When a child has gait and weight-bearing issues, parents and pediatricians need to look at the rest of the body first. There will be muscular and structural clues as to the altered tensions throughout the body. The birth history will be positive with multiple physical signs; there is almost always a history of multiple traumas, falls, and injuries in childhood. The child's collarbones may not be straight, and will rather be slightly curved. A consequence of curving at the collarbones is that the spaces at the base of the neck between the trapezius muscles, called the thoracic outlet, are narrowed. I find this commonly in children who have fallen multiple times in toddlerhood.

Ankle pronation and flat feet are essentially the same clinical entity—two sides of the same coin. They are just viewed from a different perspective. In ankle pronation, the ligaments are so loose that the ankles turn in and the full weight load of the body cannot be borne by the medial arch of the feet. In flat feet, the arches are weak and cannot support the weight load of the body. The conventional approach to treatment of flat feet is arch support and shoe inserts. Although benign and cost effective, arch supports are by definition another form of bracing. Bracing, in general, is a quick fix; this approach does not answer the question of why the feet cannot dissipate force (the truncal weight load). In the upright human posture, our trunk sits atop the pelvis and the hips. When we walk, our hips swing (rotate). Our knees bend and the knee cartilage (meniscus) cushions some of the force transmitted from the hips. The flexibility and compliance of tissues allow for dissipation of force by the time it gets to the feet; in other words, we should have enough support. I propose that the problem isn't so much in the feet or ankles, and suggest that we look along the length of the legs, all the way up into the sacroiliac joint, and perhaps also look at old past history of head injury.

For example: AC is a 40-year-old male who consulted me for sleep apnea. He was diagnosed in the last 6 months and was given a CPAP machine, but it was ruining his personal life and he wanted to be free of it. In his childhood, he experienced a blunt force trauma to the head. He had multiple falls on his tailbone, mostly acquired during skiing. As an adult male, he has been physically active in soccer and parkour. He also has flat feet which require arch supports. His osteopathic treatment lasted one hour, by the end of which, we both could feel that he felt better. Yet for the next several nights, he was miserable. Even the lowest setting on the CPAP made his ears feel like they were going to burst. Without it he could not sleep restfully; with it, he was miserable. The tensions in his body from head to toes are changing. By the end of the week, the flat feet he has had all his life began to change. He now has arches.

The lessons in this case are many. This one treatment resulted in multiple dramatic physiologic and structural changes. His case is fairly uncomplicated; he is the rare patient who has not had a car accident or surgeries. In his entire life, his most significant medical diagnosis was sleep apnea. I believe his apnea is a physiologic decompensation from years of head to toe structural tension imbalance. He came to me fairly early in his treatment; if he had had apnea for 2 or 3 years, I believe it would have taken two to three visits to effect a positive change. That the flat feet were an old problem carried over since childhood gave him the impression that his structure was a permanent problem with no solution. That the flat feet were resolved so quickly on the first visit implies that tensions can still be corrected, no matter how old. The fact that he has not had any surgery whatsoever is contributory to his immediate response. The body is able to manage and balance its own tensions *only* after the reduction of external vectors.

Pigeon Toe

All tissues in the body, especially the muscles and bones, are covered with an outer layer. In general, this covering is named after the tissue which it surrounds. For example, the lining on the outside of bone is called periosteum; for muscles, the covering is named endomysium, perimysium, and epimysium. These encasing layers, which line the muscle cell, muscle bundle, and muscle, all blend into tendon, which attaches to the bone through blending with the lining of the bone. All of this connected tissue is referred to by osteopaths as a "fascial sleeve" (I like to call it the "tissue pantyhose"). Every tissue in the body has an outer lining, and during trauma, this "sleeve" can get caught. Its restriction causes tension and pain, and osteopathic treatment helps to smooth it out. In children, as they attempt to grow and elongate, the soft tissue can get caught, resulting in tension. Regardless of where the tissue gets held up—the hip, the knee, or the ankle—it can cause the leg to turn in.

Pigeon toe is a term describing the inward pointing of the feet or toes while walking. If we watch closely, we can trace upward to where the tension lies. Is it at the ankles? Do both turn in? Is there a history of sprained ankles? Can we trace the tension up toward one or both knees? If there is tension in the knees, we can most definitely trace it further up, into the sacroiliac joints and low back.

I see these cases periodically. Conventionally, there is nothing to be done for these patients. Patients are not offered a surgical correction. The problem is one of soft tissue strain around the ankle, which can be traced back up to the area around the hip and sacroiliac joint. I would suggest that old traumas and injuries cause soft tissue restrictions.

I can only come to this conclusion because my pediatric patients usually improve the same day of treatment. They are then instructed to return at the next growth spurt, when the foot will turn in again.

CROSS EYE

Strabismus is a condition of "misalignment" of the eyes. It is one of the more common eye conditions in childhood. Eye conditions generally distress parents greatly. Esotropia, the inward turning of the eye is more common than the outward turning of an eye. The conventional approach is the conservative option: patching first, and, if the problem does not correct itself, surgery is considered by specialists in the field of ophthalmology. Eye movements are controlled by muscles external to the eye. Most ophthalmologists do not consider the possibility that changes can be attained through vision therapy exercises for those muscles. Even more difficult to comprehend, for both allopaths and osteopaths practicing conventional medicine, is the possibility of relieving tension in those muscles to ameliorate conditions with vision disturbances.

AC is a 5-year-old little girl who came to me for help with her strabismus (see Figure 16 in the photo insert). Her ophthalmologist had been pressing for surgery, and her mother had refused. Her traumatic history is that at 9 months of age, a cold iron fell on the right side of her head. She has not had any intervention. We freed up the compressive vector of the trauma from 5 years ago. The restriction in growth of the soft tissues from the traumatic force was lifted; as a result, the freed up tissues try to balance and adapt the "new" (but really old) freedom and tensions it had prior to the trauma. That one trauma in infancy has affected the development of her face in a variety of ways:

1. The shape of her face is narrow and elongated.

2. Her forehead is narrow, high, and flat.

3. The distance from the outer edge of her eyes to her temples is shortened.

4. The left upper eyelid is larger.

5. The distance between her right upper and lower eyelid is shorter.

6. The distance between the middle of her nose out to her cheek is shorter on the right.

7. The creases between her nose and lip are long and deep.

8. Her lips are thin and the lip line is long.

Even 5 years later, cranial osteopathy can help. Since we achieved changes, can we reasonably conclude that the force of that trauma has been sitting in those tissues, waiting to be unloaded? Precisely unloaded, the changes are near instantaneous (see Figure 17 in the photo insert). She needed 12 cranial osteopathic treatments, after which she was sent back to do vision therapy with a developmental vision optometrist. The results were outstanding. She needed 60 vision therapy sessions over the course of 16 months. She started out with no depth perception (stereopsis), to developing good depth perception. Her parents noted that her reading speed has increased, her handwriting has improved, and homework is easier. She is also more coordinated, with improved behavior and greater awareness of depth.

KN came to me for help with her eye. She had begged her mother to take her to someone who could fix her eye, which struck me as unusual. Children with esotropia, or any kind of structural strain, usually do not complain, because they are not aware of this being an "altered" state of tensions. One-and-a-half years ago, the left eye started to turn in. There was no history of blunt force trauma. The mother took her to an ophthalmologist who patched the eye. In the last 6 months, the right eye started to turn in significantly (see the first photo in Figure 18 in the photo insert). She was not getting results, and the family was adamant about not doing surgery. They took her to a chiropractor for several visits, to no avail. They took her to a vision therapy optometrist who suggested cranial osteopathy. Other than the eye, the same subtle clues in facial asymmetry are present:

1. The upper eyelid on the left is larger.

2. The distance from the center of her nose to the outside of her cheek is shorter on the right.

3. The right jawline is a tad more curved.

4. The right face/cheek is smaller.

With KN, the subtle asymmetries would not be noticed, and some people would disagree that these asymmetries are even there. The physical exam showed tensions from head to toe. She also had a large neck spasm on the right.

The lessons to learn from KN are several. We did not get instantaneous eye correction after one visit. Was it because I was imprecise and could not get it all reduced? After all, I do not know the traumatic cause. Whatever the original strain, someone else, another practitioner had already tried to address it. If someone else has done structural work, it is too difficult to try to decipher the original findings from partially treated ones. In cases such as these, we do what the body allows and wait for change. It took four visits for change to occur (see the second photo in Figure 18 in the photo insert).

NT was brought to me by his mother for cosmetic concerns over his left eyelid. His eyelids were noticeably asymmetric. As an infant he had had surgery to correct esotropia in the right eye. Again, the same types of symptoms were observed:

1. The right eye appears smaller.

2. The tip of the nose seems to be deviating to the right.

3. The right cheek appears to be narrow and smaller.

Surgery scars up connective tissue, and I generally do not offer too much hope of getting any changes. NT also has a congenital condition of his left foot. His mother refused surgery. When I treat NT's feet, he walks easier and lighter; he does not "thunk" around the house in heavy feet. His feet hurt, but when he is treated, his pain is relieved. NT is a good case of the soft tissue response of surgery, which is usually permanence of tissue strain at the local level. The lessons here are twofold: 1) that surgery scars up connective tissue sleeves, after which not much can be done (when compared to the previous two severe cases); and 2) even in this patient, where surgery was deemed "necessary" for a foot condition found at birth, we found that we were still able to reduce the pain and improve function (see Figure 19 in the photo insert).

Every physician is asked by patients and parents what they would do for themselves or friends and family. And in every field of medicine, I believe that most physicians treat their patients the way they would like to be treated. I have my own issues with my eye, and my experiences in dealing with these issues are an excellent example of the osteopathic perspective, and how we would take care of ourselves.

LH: For 5 years after the birth of my children, I experienced pain, achiness and poor vision in my left eye. It would intermittently ache, which implies no permanent injury. I knew the health of my eyes was not at risk. The general achiness was not internal to the eye; it felt external and structural. I knew conventional ophthalmology would advise corrective lenses, but it wasn't until I did more advanced cranial coursework that I realized that I had a cranial strain, one which had resulted from a traumatic dental procedure. In my early thirties, I had my wisdom teeth removed. The upper left wisdom tooth had a root that was hooked, and during the two hours it took for the dentist to surgically extract it he pulled, torqued, and yanked the root, resulting in three vectors of injury in at least two planes of motion. When procedures are done where force is applied to the upper teeth, the patient generally suffers ill effects afterward. This is because the roof of the mouth, viewed from above, is really the other side of the base of the skull. When the dentist was yanking on the tooth, he was really pulling out the bony orbital floor of my left eye. Do I blame the dentist? No; how was he supposed to know? Do I blame me? I should have at least caught on sooner than the 5 years it took me, suffering all the while. After all, we are repeatedly reminded that the placement of the head and neck during dental procedures is unnatural with respect to how our mouth and jaw should function. Worse, an extended period of time for a procedure does cause strain. I had left eye symptoms, and I had previously had a left wisdom tooth pulled. These are not coincidental, but directly related; it just took time and two pregnancies to manifest.

Five years and six traditional osteopathic physician colleagues later, my left eye experiences periods of good achiness. I can almost describe it as "un-aching," retreating from the way it used to ache terribly. I am undergoing vision therapy myself and it is helping my brain re-pattern and relearn what used to be my normal binocular vision.

In summary, from the four cases gathered here, several points can be made:

1. Prior intervention means less effective osteopathy.

2. Ideally, it is best to treat when trauma occurs; but even old strain patterns are treatable.

CONSTIPATION

As a pediatrician, at every well-child exam, we ask about daily bowel movements. I often tell parents, "A poopy baby is a happy baby." In the natural state, a fully breastfed baby will have a bowel movement as often as every feed. Some systems tend to be a little slower, but as long as an infant makes one bowel movement a day, they are generally happy. Some systems can be a little sluggish, and they catch up in the following days without any intervention. Pathologically sluggish systems are diagnosed as constipation. When there is straining at stool, this is constipation. When there is an urge that does not easily result in a product, this is constipation. Having hard dry stools or pellet-like stools is constipation. When a child needs intervention with juice, laxatives, stool softeners, or enemas, know that these are merely quick fixes that result in evacuation of the bowels. The normal state of the bowels is sequential muscular contractions of the gut tube (called peristalsis) that results in a bowel movement.

In the earliest part of human development, the gut starts off as a hose from the mouth to the anus. Food goes in the one end and waste moves out the other. Movement of food through this tube should be fairly smooth. A fair analogy for movement of the bowels is water running through a hose. In the gut, we have a soft solid that needs to be propelled forward. Over the counter medications such as bulk laxatives (psyllium husk), osmotic laxatives (milk of magnesia, MiraLax) and stool softeners serve to change the nature of that solid to semisolid, or even a liquid. Minerals and other types of oils coat the solid, greasing it up and easing the movement of the solid. I favor the senna teas and laxatives that mildly irritate and stimulate the gut for muscular contractions. The irritation also causes fluid to enter the gut to soften the stool.

About 10 percent of children have constipation. Ninety percent of those children have functional constipation that responds to oral interventions. Chronic intervention does not answer the question of why this person's system is not working correctly. From an osteopathic mechanical medical perspective, we look at the gut tube as a hose that hangs down from the middle of our head. Along the length of the hose on the back side, the hose is anchored to our body, deeply and internally. On the front side, the hose is fairly free so that some movement is allowed. This "muscular hose" is also designed and packaged to fit nicely. There is a balance of anchoring to provide stability, but there needs to be relative freedom for movement. The soap-on-a-rope concept holds here, in that the gut can twist and get stuck.

Conventional medicine recognizes the extreme twisting called volvulus. When symptoms of pain, vomiting, and abdominal distention worsen, it suggests that the blood supply is kinked, and there is concern that tissue may die. This is a surgical emergency. This twisting is understood to happen, but how or why it happens is not well understood. These issues are addressed after the fact and dealt with it at the time it presents.

In the day-to-day pediatric setting, I see a milder version of the twisting and kinking of the hose. Mechanically, these are a result of rolling off the bed or couch, followed by the impact on the floor or carpet, which sets up a mild traumatic twisting strain. A child may not be symptomatic with one fall; it usually takes multiple mild little falls, in different directions and different types to slow down the gut. As the child's body attempts to grow and elongate, it is then that the gut becomes more sluggish. The prior traumatic tensions are now further strained in multiple directions as the abdominal cavity tries to stretch out in three dimensions. As muscular contractions try to move the food along the gut, the contractions are no longer smooth and well-coordinated. The bowels' movements are now slowed.

This is RW, who we discussed in Part II (page 31). We had just finished a treatment when his mother remarked at how different he looked. I had done a lot of structural work on his shoulders, and had not expected much facial or jaw change. The first picture in Figure 20 (see the photo insert), was taken by his mother's phone a week prior to his appointment. The second picture shows the remarkable improvement we saw after his treatment. Today, he appears more mature and handsome; less elfin, with his chin less pointy and his eyes less narrowed. For any patient (if I want to open up the face and jaw), I always treat at the shoulder and collarbone. These structural findings and changes correlate with his initial presentation.

The initial reason for his visit was chronic constipation. The complaint was that he would sit in the bathroom straining. His bowel movements were as infrequent as every 7 days. His history of trauma includes multiple falls and rolling off of the bed in the first 2 years of life. Upon examining him, I could detect a rolling strain pattern, which can often be observed in the physical body and lie of the patient. In a relaxed state, while the patient is comfortable, the head is often more likely to be positioned to one side. The chest will be rotated to the same side. The hip on that side will be more open to that side. The leg and foot will tend to point to the same side. The consequence of rolling to one side is that there is now asymmetry of the sides of the body. One side of the body tends to be more "open" and the opposite side will be more "closed." The "open" side will function fairly well; it is the opposing "closed" side where the patient has some dysfunction. Often, the patient will state that one side of their body is weaker.

After de-rotating and balancing his muscular tensions his mom reported that the bowel movement improved to every 3 days. On follow-up visits we reviewed his traumatic history and it turns out that he was in his car seat as a 4-year-old child when he and his mother were rear-ended. Upon hearing that, I proceeded to treat him for rear-end collision vectors. His mother reported that within the week, his bowels had become normal and daily, without straining.

CHAPTER 13

Adolescence
(10–18 years)

ADOLESCENCE IS a period of both great structural changes and great hormonal changes. These hormonal changes contribute to skin changes, but also compound with high velocity strains, leading to an exacerbation in a teenager's normal condition. Rapid growth also strains the growing skeletal and muscular systems, and can lead to complaints of pain.

ACNE

One of the hallmarks of puberty is the appearance of acne. In response to an upsurge in sex hormones, oil glands and sweat glands become active. Dead skin cells and oils clog pores, and bacteria on the skin begin to thrive on those oils. The tissue response is redness and inflammation.

There are varying degrees of acne. In the most severe cases, patients are referred to dermatologists. Patients who find me are usually coming to me for different reasons, and not for their acne. The acne is incidental; they usually don't even mention it because by the time they see me, they have been to the dermatologist, have tried everything, and have given up.

My osteopathic philosophical approach is that the inflow and out-flow of the blood supply to the head, neck, and face is out of balance. The ability of the veins to drain is always affected by physical trauma. Blood is actively pumped up and into the head and neck by the heart. Drainage of blood by way of the veins is passive. When trauma occurs, kinking in both the veins and arteries occurs but alterations in flow happen in the veins. When I treat patients and reduce their traumatic injury vectors, I usually find that there was a high velocity accident in their past that has affected them. I generally instruct patients that osteopathic manipulative treatment (OMT) optimizes blood flow in and out, to and from the skin of the face, head, and neck. The balanced interchange helps to mitigate the contributions of hormones, hygiene, and genetically inherited skin tendencies.

Conventional medicine does not attribute mechanical causes to acne, other than that of blocked pores. The conventional medicine mechanical approach is to scrub off the dead cells and bacteria. In infants with splotchy cheeks and scalp, osteopathic treatment clears them up (in conjunction with formula changes). Likewise, the changes that can happen during adolescence may require other lifestyle modifications. Successful treatment usually requires commitment to slow, gradual, and consistent use of multiple approaches.

In the two case examples below, the patients showed slow changes in their acne without any other changes in their skin care regimen or dermatologist's prescription medication regimen. The results show that high velocity injuries contribute to exacerbation of the patient's natural tendencies.

EP has been my patient, on and off, for about 10 years. I first met her when she was a teenager and her family sought help for her chronic sinus infections. Prior to coming to see me, she had already had two sinus surgeries. We started treatments and since then, she has not needed any more surgeries. She does not need chronic nasal steroids or chronic oral medications. When she gets really bad, it is because she came in too late, at which point she needs antibiotics and an osteopathic manipulative treatment (OMT). I saw her infrequently in her teen years. Now that she is in her mid-twenties, the stress from work and poor diet are bringing her in more frequently with her sinus tendencies.

In her teens, her complexion was clear. The outbreak of her acne is more of an adult onset. As our rapport improved with her maturity, I recently found out that she was involved in a rear-end collision when she was 8 years old. She then had her two surgeries back to back when she was 10 years old. Most conventional pediatricians would not attribute causation, much less a relationship, between these two major events in her early adolescence. I would suggest that they are directly related, and would propose that the one car accident destabilized her allergic tendencies and structurally contributed to her inability to drain her sinuses effectively. She had already demonstrated allergy and sinus tendencies in the years prior. The high velocity rear-end collision destabilized her. From that point on, the infections increased and were more difficult to control, until one day her sinuses were close to bursting with pus. It took several years and almost twenty visits for her to improve, after which she needed to come in less frequently. As her sinuses improved, she developed moderate acne. She reports to me that she continues to mostly sleep on her belly (see the prior section on sleep positioning). To the traditional osteopathic physician, this is all part and parcel of the same *traumatic derailment syndrome.*

In this set of before and after photos (see Figure 21 in the photo insert), she is not on any medication for the acne (topical or oral). Note the change in the redness of the acne lesions. Her forehead is less shiny and less inflamed. This whole visit was focused primarily on the reduction of the traumatic vectors of the rear-end collision in her legs, hips, back, shoulders, and neck. I also reduced some of the soft tissue tensions of the intubated head, neck, face, jaw, shoulder, sternum, ribs, and the left intubated hip. Even though she came in for complaints unrelated to her acne, I took these photos to demonstrate that when a traumatic event occurs, it happens to the whole body. If, in undoing the vectors of a trauma, we get results, we can conclude that that trauma must have contributed to that "disease" state.

SE is a patient who was brought in by his mother for a consultation of structure. As a newborn infant, he was intubated to help him breathe. An image search for the terms "pediatric ET tube" will show the tool that pediatricians, neonatologists, and pediatric anesthesiologists use to control the infant airway and to help them breathe. A search for "pediatric laryngoscope" will reveal what we use to assist the placement of the ET tube. This very first procedure was important in saving his life, and he was intubated for a total of 2 days.

Later, as a toddler and young child, he was involved in several car accidents (two rear-end collisions and one T-bone collision), all of which when taken together have contributed to his suffering and have manifested as acne and his mechanically inefficient and exhausting posture (seen in the photo on the left). Before treatment, his head and neck are pitched forward and his upper back is excessively rounded (see Figure 22a in the photo insert).

Over the course of five visits in 2 months, without changing any of his skin or antibiotic regimens, his skin is much clearer (see the photos in Figure 22b in the photo insert). By October, his head and neck were eased back and his back is a straighter line. His mom reports that his thyroid labs are also improved. His global improvements in posture, skin, gait, and thyroid hormones are typical of traditional osteopathic treatments. SE states that he can tell when his body starts to feel heavy, which is a sign that he needs to return for another visit. After just five visits for a lifetime of strain and high velocity soft tissue injuries, he does not need to rely on me to tell him when he needs treatment. He can feel it, and trusts himself to decide when to come back. I generally instruct all of my patients to learn to sense their bodies, so that when changes happen they can tell much sooner whether they need to come in.

SCOLIOSIS

Scoliosis is a complex structural condition with so many attendant variables that it deserves its own book. In general, scoliosis refers to a condition in which the spine is not straight. There are natural curves in the human spine when observed from the side; viewed from the back, the vertebral column can be thought of as blocks, stacked on top of each other. The intervertebral discs are very much like cushions in between each block of bone. Each and every individual vertebra and disc above and below should all stack up nicely and fairly straight.

There are several types of curves. There are single C curves, double S curves, and compensatory curves, some of which include a worsening of the roundness (kyphosis) of the upper back, some with flattening of the upper back. Part of the side-bending in a scoliosis includes rotation of the segments.

In a textbook used for training in general pediatrics, scoliosis is defined as a complex, three-dimensional abnormality of the spine. The diagnosis is one of exclusion, in that all other factors need to be ruled out. In idiopathic scoliosis, the cause is unknown, but likely to include genetic and environmental factors. Although genetic mechanisms have been proposed, no gene has been identified: "*Abnormalities identified in connective tissue, muscle, and bone appear to be secondary*".[48]

This last statement is quoted verbatim; the special emphasis is mine. It is obvious and grossly observable that in idiopathic scoliosis there are bending or curving vectors in all three planes of the human spine. I disagree with this and believe the converse to be the truth. The human spine bends and curves, but it does so because the forces locked in the surrounding connective tissue, muscle, and bone holding the scoliosis in place are *primary*. Conventionally, when a patient is diagnosed with scoliosis, it is usually because there is a persistent pain. The doctor checks the back and finds the curve. If it is mild, they are sent to physical therapy, given stretches, and told to stay active. More moderate to severe scoliosis is conventionally addressed by bracing or surgery.

Two studies worth discussing show the long-term follow-up for procedures for scoliosis. The first study followed patients who decide to brace. The goal of bracing is not to cure, nor is it treatment to improve the curve; rather, it is intended to prevent curve *progression*. At the end of the study, 60 percent to 90 percent of patients had moderate to severe pain. Those who had surgery had a slightly lower quality of life (9 percent).[49]

The second study followed patients who had surgery with placement of a Harrington Rod. This surgery straightens the spine by placing a rigid metal rod along the spinal column. The author of the study admits that there is limited derotation of the segments. At the 4-year post-operation evaluation, two-thirds of patients showed *increasing* rib prominence.[50] The surgery may have stabilized the rotational component in a third of the patients, but the remaining progression of the rotational vectors tells me that the forces in the underlying cause have not been addressed.

It is my opinion that the osteopathic philosophy is far more elegant. When conventional doctors talk about scoliosis and rotation of a vertebral segment, they tend to focus their attention on the most pronounced area of the curves. The tendency is to think of that area as rotating and involving those segments around an axis that runs along the column at each level. I see the rotation as more of a twist or a spiral strain. If we step back and examine the whole backside of a patient with idiopathic scoliosis, it should include a view of the back of the skull and the sacrum (the bone between the buttocks). Often, these patients will have asymmetries from the head down through the trunk and into the tailbone. From the back view, one ear may appear to be more forward, toward the face. The other ear may appear lowered to that shoulder. Viewed from the front, there will be corresponding facial asymmetries. One brow may be higher, one side of the jaw may be tighter, and one eye may be smaller. When we examine the sacrum at the level of the waist, it might have a tendency to be more rotated to one side. One hip might appear higher. So the spiral vector is a total truncal twisting strain. Let us ask the question, "When in the history of a human being do we acquire this type of strain?"

In the course of human embryonic development, there is plenty of room for the spine to grow fairly straight, symmetrical, and unimpeded. By 4 months of gestation, the baby is larger and mothers can begin to feel fetal movements. This implies reciprocal tensions and a dynamic interaction between the baby's push and the maternal uterine stretch. If the baby moves fairly freely, then we can be more assured of there being enough room for unimpeded symmetrical movement and growth.

One of the most influential periods in fetal development contributing to later scoliosis is the birth process. It lays the structural foundation for the tendency toward scoliosis and augments the genetic contributory factors. In the birth process, the baby does not shoot out smooth and straight like a torpedo out of the birth canal. The baby is propelled by uterine contractions down a relatively narrow opening that should be compliant and expand with contractions. In order to accommodate the bony maternal hips and muscles of the pelvis, the baby has to spiral. With the head and whole body compressed, all the soft tissues from head to toe experience this spiraling strain. If there is a problem somewhere along the path, another strain may be placed over the first. Two common additional overlying strains are those caused by forceps or a vacuum. In the case of forceps, the cheeks are clamped and the face compressed from the sides. When a vacuum is used, it may seem less problematic for the infant, but it comes with its own share of negative forces. Using a different method to assist in the extraction of a stuck baby results in our having traded compressive vectors for shearing, hyperextending, and potentially twisting strains.

The birth itself is the primary underlying spiral vector strain that is embedded in the soft tissue, pre-connective tissue, pre-muscle, and pre-bone tissues from head to tailbone. It is also very possible that there may be a primary familial genetic tendency to idiopathic scoliosis. In the first year of life, the physical body is still unformed, so this spiral strain is not evident. For example, a Slinky with one or two caught coils is not as noticeable when it is collapsed and small. However, as it is stretched, visually, mechanically, and functionally those coils impinge more and more. The difficulty is proportional to the number of caught coils (vectors) and the speed with which the stretch is attempted (growth velocity is greatest at puberty). Add in other difficult birth circumstances such as a bigger, later baby; a cord around the neck; or worse, breech position with multiple attempts at turning; and the strains around the head and neck are already compounded. Add in a rambunctious early childhood, roughhousing with siblings, early sports, and accidents and all of these strains start to add up. They play a more prominent role if they are acquired earlier in the formative stages of the musculoskeletal system.

KK has functional scoliosis. KK broke her ankle at 6 years of age, and 4 years later at her annual physical, to my surprise, she had developed a scoliosis. Her mother reminded me about the left ankle, which had required two rounds of physical therapy. The muscles are tight and contract the leg so that it appears shorter, which causes her hip to drop when she stands or walks (see the first photo in Figure 23 in the photo insert). The differing leg lengths cause a downward tilt of the sacral base (at the waist) on the side of the shorter leg. The tilt drags down on the side of the back and causes a corresponding twist that is transmitted to her upper back. While she is sitting down, her trunk is stable and shoulders are level. The pelvic tilt from the short leg leads to an unstable spinal column. She only needed two visits before the scoliosis, the short leg, and the pelvic tilt were resolved (see the second photo in Figure 23 in the photo insert).

MM: The first photo in Figure 24 (in the photo insert) shows a very mild thoracic scoliosis. MM responded well after one treatment (see the second photo in Figure 24 in the photo insert). There is still a residual asymmetry in the shoulders and tightness of the right side of the trunk. MM is very active in sports and she needs several more visits to truly free the tensions and strains. She was happy enough with her results and she did not come back.

NC is a teenager who has the beginnings of scoliosis, with a strong family history of scoliosis pointing to a genetic component: both her father and grandmother have a scoliosis. When NC started with her scoliosis, we decided to wait and observe it. As it worsened, I referred her to an orthopedic specialist. They had a consultation and, given that the scoliosis was at a severe 47 degrees, the specialist recommended immediate surgery—bracing was not even offered. Both her father and grandmother had been offered the option of surgery to address their scoliosis, but only the grandmother had opted to have a rod inserted along her spine. Her father remains very active today, but her grand-mother experiences chronic pain as a result of her surgery. Because of these two extreme outcomes resulting from the different therapeutic choices, they opted not to do surgery for NC. They chose to go to a chiropractor who was a specialist in exercises for scoliosis. They did not see much improvement with her spine, and she began having osteopathic manipulative treatments with me. For many visits, I did not notice any improvement. On one visit, I tried several stretches and exercises. After each set of movements, I would recheck her back, with no results. Then, one day she came in complaining of back pain. Generally, idiopathic scoliosis patients don't complain of pain. That she did so was quite unusual, but she had just returned from tennis camp. I asked how long she had played tennis. She answered that she had played since she was 6 years old. Her back was so severely twisted, it was frightening. I pondered the possibility that tennis was exacerbating a preexisting genetic tendency. I took her out into the hall and asked her to pretend to play tennis for me. As I watched her, I became horri-fied. She had the most bizarre, ungraceful left handed serve I have ever seen. She has never had lessons, and to say the least, she has very poor form. At the end of the serve, she had a significant rightward twist—her scoliosis twist.

I instructed her on "unserving" with the left hand, and then serving with the right, recalling Dr. Miller's admonition to "engage" the strain before "disengaging" it. The logic of this osteopathic approach is ele-gant and simple. It is not at all aggressive, nor even assertive. All of the exercises I had previously tried with her failed because they were imprecise. On this day, we found the exacerbating cause and tested it by precisely reducing the vectors using multiple motions. The result was instantaneous resolution of her back pain for that day. This result proved the theory. I instructed her to do these exercises as often as she could remember to do so, as often as she breathes, for the rest of her life. To be more precise, the sum total of the force of the wacky left handed serve accumulated over the past 6 years needed to be unloaded. If she is diligent and does her "un-exercise" regularly and consistently, she may not need to do it for the rest of her life. But like most teens and most people, we forget. I suspect that after a period of consistency, she will stop. The total torsional, twisting force will only be partially reduced. Unfortunately, I have no follow-up as she has not returned.

There is one final learning point in the case of NC. Previously, she had no pain to guide us as to causation. She went to multiple specialists and her parents made informed choices about how best to care for her. Even with me, there were many visits, with only slight improvements. There were multiple trials and attempts and failures at finding the precise movements, stretches, rotations, and de-rotations. Most people give up the search for answers. It took several years to finally figure out the puzzle. Unfortunately, a case of idiopathic scoliosis like NC will likely never show up again. The next one may be completely different. It may be a teenager, a top rank national fencer, or an Olympics bound swimmer—all of whom will have different clues to decipher to find the final answer.

GROWING PAINS

In infancy, most growth occurs in the head; in early childhood, most growth occurs in the trunk; and in adolescents, most growth occurs in the long bones. It is most common in the adolescent period (and especially in the pubertal growth spurts) that kids complain of pain in the leg, often in or around the shins. Parents and pediatricians alike ascribe this to growth, or growing pains. Most children complain at night and after a long day of activity. Parents mostly feel helpless and can only offer massaging or ibuprofen. Because this is a temporary condition, and not serious, the majority of kids are left to suffer with their pain. Conventional medicine has little to offer in terms of explanation or alleviation. The traditional osteopathic approach offers treatment to alleviate the pain. I feel that the pain isn't so much in the growing bones, but rather, the growth is attempting to stretch out kinks, twists, and compression strains in the fascial sleeves of the tissues of the legs. The sleeve that surrounds the bone called the periosteum is known to be sensitive. Most conventional doctors do not deal very much with the soft tissue lining around muscle or periosteum. Osteopathy reduces tensions in these connective tissues, and patients typically respond well to these treatments In fact, my patients usually get up and walk out of my office without pain.

ANXIETY

In the conventional medical system, anxiety in teens and adult patients is generally dealt with using a pharmaceutical approach, either prescribed by a primary care doctor or, for complex cases, by a psychiatrist or neurologist.

I often see teenage and adult patients with anxiety. The mechanical causes and presentations vary. When patients complain of anxiety that starts in the chest, of not being able to breathe which causes panic to set in, I usually look to the back for scoliosis. With a twist going through the middle of the back, the rib tension and relationship between the ribs are altered and asymmetric. To breathe, the ribs need to lift up symmetrically in an inhalation and sink down in exhalation. If there is a scoliosis in the middle back, the ribs do not lift up evenly, air flow is inefficient and tensions can be altered in the diaphragm. The diaphragm is a large muscle that separates our chest cavity from the abdominal cavity. Its rhythmic downward contraction creates negative pressure in the chest cavity that allows air to move into the airway. With tension and strain, or spasms from a trauma, breathing may be impaired just enough that the patient is distressed, but not enough to be life-threatening. When patients report their symptoms and no other medical causes are found, patients are told that it is all "in their head."

For the traditional osteopathic physician, anxiety is a real clinical entity with mechanical causes. With or without the breathing component in a patient's story, I will look to the head. I will ask about head trauma, not just recent injuries in the several months prior to the onset of the anxiety, but all the way back to infancy. High velocity head trauma shocks the whole nervous system. After the superficial bruises and scratches heal, the brain matter will still have difficulty dealing with the jolt.

Cranial osteopathy is highly specialized, and most conventional M.D.s do not believe that there is actually minor freedom of movement between the parts of the skull. Sutures, the joints in the skull where the bony plates meet, become jammed and locked up after a trauma. The tension relationship of all the bony skull parts is altered. These subtle relationships of bone, brain, and tissue matter in the day-to-day complexity of living and breathing, and also affect how we sleep and how we function neurologically. The patient is usually not aware of how heavy their head feels. They do not realize that they don't sleep well. After a cranial osteopathic treatment to undo the traumatic vectors of injury, the restrictions at the bony sutures free up. The patient feels instantaneous relief. They are now aware that their head is lighter and can move their neck a little more freely.

When blunt force trauma is not present in the history of an anxious teen or adult, I look for repetitive, low-force stress injury. In the teenager, there is often a history of orthodontic work or worse, an intubation for a medically necessary procedure. Both types of procedures will alter the tensions in the neck, jaw, face, and head. Both cause a change in the positioning of the frontal lobe, the part of the brain that sits just behind the forehead. A cranial osteopathic treatment to correct this positioning reduces tensions in the sutures, in the bones, and in the brain. The reduced tensions allow the patient to settle and calm down. Patients over time need less medication. Parents often observe an immediate relaxation in the teenager's posture and facial expression.

BEHAVIORAL ISSUES

Parents often attribute behavioral issues in their teenager to the stresses of school, peers, and hormonal changes. Very rarely are parents aware of trauma affecting their teen's behavior. If the behavior change is abrupt, I ask about any recent injuries, specifically a head injury. If the behavioral changes are slow and over a period of time, I would suspect a repetitive stress injury (dental or intubation) affecting sleep. Non-restful sleep (what I call "false sleep") can be evidenced by tossing and turning with sheets, pillows, arms, and legs askew. The patient is unable to go into deep restful REM sleep, and does not wake up refreshed. The teenager does not feel good, yet they do not *know* that they don't feel good. They end up snapping at people and are quick to lose their temper. Over time, schoolwork suffers and teachers and classmates start to notice.

I was treating Maya, whose family lived two hours away. She told me that just the other day, her son Jacob was not careful in watching his step and walked into a glass door. As they live far away, and coming in for a visit is difficult with his school schedule, I told her to, "Wait until he gets mean." Two weeks later, they both came in and she tells me, "You were right! Out of the blue he just snapped!" In general, Jacob is a nice, mild-mannered, easy-going kid. But in light of the recent head trauma, both parents decided it was time for him to come in. It took one visit to bring him back to his normal self.

In teenagers, whose neck, head, face, and jaw tensions have been altered by procedures (especially intubations), behavioral changes usually happen several months later. This is especially insidious because of the delayed effect; parents and patients do not realize how altered they are. Even my established patients and parents who already know about my osteopathic work forget that trauma can affect their teen's behavior. They only bring their teenager in as a last resort. They try talking to their teen and to the teachers, they evaluate his homework; they try to understand, but to no avail. When I ask what happened in between the last time I saw the patient and now, there is often some procedure or trauma at the root of things.

MH is such a case (see the section under swayback in the photo insert). I did not know this child as previously having this structure. A bright kid, she enjoys school and generally does well. By the time of this visit, she was in danger of failing for the year. I attributed the physical and behavioral changes to her prior intubation. She felt immediately better after the treatment. I gave her exercises to do for the rest of her life.

CHAPTER 14

Chronic Conditions at Any Age

AUTISM

AUTISM IS a complex neurologic and developmental disorder that presents with varying degrees of symptoms. Autistic patients have difficulties in speech, communication, and awareness of self and others. Social interactions are affected, from a mild to a severe degree. In more severe cases there may be self-injurious behavior or seizure disorders. The symptoms are so variable in presentation that they are described as falling on a spectrum: autism spectrum disorder (ASD). Children may be diagnosed as early as infancy or as late in childhood as 3 years of age. At this time, there is no identifiable gene or direct cause for autism. The current conventional medical understanding is that there is a genetic component that, combined with various environmental factors, influences the development of autism.

From my clinical experience, I have always felt autism to be traumatic brain injury *first*, as a primary derailment. Then, further subsequent insults: another head injury, multiple minor injuries, or a vaccine reaction. The accumulation of factors determines the degree of severity once it manifests. With each family I interview, there is always, first, a difficult pregnancy or birth. The infant seems to be doing well until another injury, either a car accident, a fall or a head injury.

In adults, we know that following head injuries, patients with traumatic brain injuries have problems with recognizing emotions from facial expressions.[51] In children, we know that shaken babies have poor neurologic outcomes. In one small study, in 25 babies followed for 59 months, 64 percent of shaken baby syndrome (SBS) patients have speech and language difficulties, including autism.[52]

It is only recently that more research has clarified and strengthened my views based on my clinical observations and treatment results. A long, difficult birth causes infant head compression over a period of time. When the contractions are irregular and not strong enough, Pitocin is used to "augment" the contractions. The difficulty of the birth, which itself causes significant compressive loading of the infant head, is further compounded by this use of Pitocin, which is supposed to help move the baby along faster, at the cost of putting more pressure on the infant skull. Researchers looking at birth records in North Carolina and comparing them to an educational database found an association between Pitocin-assisted births and autism.[53]

As described in Chapters 2 and 3, compressive loads on the infant skull, when viewed by the traditional osteopathic physician, are seen to affect the drainage of veins. It is a fact in human anatomy that blood flow *into* the cranium is active via the pumping of the heart. Blood flow *out* of the head is passive, by way of the veins. In other words, there is no active pumping mechanism to ensure blood flow out of the brain. If both inflow and outflow were controlled and regulated, compressive loads on the skull or acute head injury would not be as serious or consequential. Researchers in China doing blood flow mapping in the brains of autistic patients found decreased blood flow in areas of the lower brain white matter around the cranial base.[54]

Other autism researchers have found that in autistic patients, the white matter growth in the brain is disproportionate.[55] The grey matter in humans is what separates us from lower primates. The white matter is considered "supportive" in this role. The white matter consists of multiple types of cells that are responsible for immunity, neuroprotection, and neuro-destructive roles. Mostly called microglia, these cells chew up sick or damaged brain cells.[56] These are the "garbage men" in the brain. Where there is an abundance of these "garbage men," it is sensible to assume an abundance of "garbage" is present as well. Why would there be more sick and damaged brain cells? When cells are starved of nutrients or oxygen delivered by blood flow, it implies that the flow is affected. The cells are groggy and bloated because they are immersed in metabolic waste from cellular respiration. The results suggest an "ongoing postnatal process".[57] I would suggest that this ongoing process is venous congestion, reflected in distended bulging veins along the scalp. I see this as redness and blood suffusion of the scalp in cranky or fussy babies that cannot suck and swallow well. If not treated, it will manifest as pain in later life, a pain that the patient likely will not recognize as abnormal. They may have frequent headaches and will not sleep as well. They are in their own world, and that world is full of hurt and suffering.

So far, one of the more promising conventional approaches is applied behavioral analysis (ABA). Applied behavioral analysis in a retrospective study of 38 children showed that with early intensive intervention, autism patients may achieve functioning in the average range.[58] Another study estimates that 3 percent to 25 percent of autistic syndrome disorder patients can recover. The proposed mechanisms of recovery include: "normalizing input by forcing attention outward or enriching the environment; promoting the reinforcement value of social stimuli; preventing interfering behaviors; mass practice of weak skills; reducing stress and stabilizing arousal. Improving nutrition and sleep quality is non-specifically beneficial." And even after "recovery," there are still "residual vulnerabilities... such as tics, depression and phobias"[59] that remain. These statements imply "asserting" (if not coercing) the patient into accepting the expectation of normal. But even after they are deemed "recovered," they are not *normal*.

I propose traditional osteopathic treatments to decompress the compressive loading of the infant cranium from a difficult augmented birth, or else the reduction of traumatic vectors of high velocity injury or blunt force trauma. My two "curative" cases involved children who were treated early and had only mild symptoms, without other serious medical problems.

Twin B was brought to me by her mother when she was 3 years old. The schoolteacher had recommended that she get an evaluation for her hand flapping behaviors. She is shy and does not have any friends. Regional Center (a state facility that diagnoses and provides autism services) diagnosed her as autistic. On physical examination, even though her head circumference measurement was normal and the shape of her head looked normal, it had the *feel* of a lopsided head. The history was consistent with the feel. She was twin B; while her sister twin A was active, kicking, and moving around in the womb, she was in a small corner of the womb, barely moving. I did cranial osteopathic treatments to reduce the lopsided feel of her cranium. Her mother noticed improvements with the hand flapping, and during sleep she appeared calmer. When the behaviors changed it meant the head was growing and getting stuck, or growing and returning to the pattern of lopsidedness. I instructed her mother to observe her, as the changes should also coincide with growth spurts, and to bring her in for treatment each time. It took 25 visits over 2 years. In her third year with Regional Center, she had a reevaluation. All supportive services were removed because she no longer had a diagnosis. Her mother reports that she is more interactive with her teacher, and she now has friends of her own. When she gets excited, she still flaps her hands but she knows she is flapping her hands and tells her mom that she can't help it. They calm her down and she is fine.

Baby H is brought to me by his parents at 2 month of age. His two brothers, ages 7 and 9, are both autistic. This time, with their third boy, his parents vowed to do everything differently. They had a home birth with no interventions or injections. I did a cranial osteopathic treatment and had them come back for a second visit. At 4 months of age, the baby demonstrated great eye contact and was smiling. I do not know whether the parents are convinced that the two cranial osteopathic treatments saved their third baby from autism, but I do believe that they are no longer so trusting of conventional medicine.

Autism is such a devastating disorder for patients and families that it deserves more space and time than I can provide. For our purposes, this discussion is intentionally narrow in order to focus on traditional osteopathy and what it can offer. My recommendation for families with autism in their history is to consider C-sections, if there is maternal history of gynecologic disorders or pelvic trauma. I would advise great flexibility to allow the obstetrician to decide on a C-section. If the delivery is vaginal and augmented, I suggest cranial osteopathic treatments when medical need arises. As with all neurologic and developmental disorders, early intervention—whether conventionally supportive or osteopathic—is key. As traumatic brain injury can occur at any time in life, I would recommend a period of rest and "settling down" before finding help with cranial osteopathic treatment.

BRONCHITIS/PNEUMONIA

Infants, children, and adults who have a tendency toward developing bronchitis and pneumonia have a problem of ventilation. Conventional medicine looks at these respiratory infections as localized infections in the respiratory system, to be treated with antibiotics and respiratory medication. This regimen is used over and over again for each and every episode. The traditional osteopathic physician sees frequent chest infections as an asynchronous total body respiratory mechanism, running from head to toe. Conventional scientific studies of respiration and the pulmonary system focus on a single diaphragm—the respiratory diaphragm. To the traditional osteopathic physician, there are three body diaphragms that contribute to effective mechanical ventilation of the entire system. Conventional medicine recognizes two of our three diaphragms as "true" diaphragms, in that they are muscles that separate body compartments. The two muscular diaphragms that are so recognized are the respiratory diaphragm and the pelvic diaphragm. Most conventional doctors (whether M.D.s or D.O.s) would have difficulty believing that the state of the pelvic diaphragm contributes in any way to respiratory status. The case below will demonstrate this connection.

Nicole is a 4-year-old mother of three children, with her youngest being 7 years old. She came to me for a follow-up after spending time in emergency care. She was diagnosed with asthmatic bronchitis and given a prescription for an antibiotic and an asthma inhaler. When I saw her, she was still coughing and was not noticeably better. It took me about 10 minutes to explain how her pregnancies and their vaginal delivery had stretched the resting length of the muscles of her pelvic floor. The looser pelvic floor diaphragm has her pelvic contents sitting lower, all of which are causing a muscular and connective tissue drag effect on the respiratory diaphragm. It took me another 5 minutes to osteopathically tighten up her pelvic floor muscles. Her breathing improved immediately. I made no changes in her medication. One year later, she informed me that since that one visit, she has gotten over her bronchitis and has not needed her inhaler.

The third diaphragm contributing to respiration and mechanical ventilation of the entire human system lies in the head. Conventional doctors will scoff at the thought. This "diaphragm" is not muscular, but is rather made of connective tissue. The brain has a lining called dura that I liken to plastic wrap. There are three layers of dura that line the brain and nerves, as well as the inner bony walls of the skull. When they fold over, they form a thick connective tissue sheath (called the falx) that separates the two hemispheres of the brain, and another one that separates the brain from the lower brain stem. This sheet of connective tissue that separates the upper brain area (supratentorium) from the lower brain area (infratentorial region) is the third, nonmuscular diaphragm called the tentorium cerebelli.

For cranial osteopaths, the tension between the two sheets balances and alternates, so that the brain and skull contents ventilate and *breathe*. The balancing act between the connective tissue sheets is part of a *cranial mechanism*. The actions of this diaphragm have to be matched up and synchronous with the actions of the other two to ventilate the entire body. It took me a long time to come to this understanding. It is the only way to effect permanent healing changes for patients with bronchitis and other respiratory difficulties.

JM is a 5-year-old boy brought to me by his mother. In his short little life he has had six pneumonias. His doctor has him on steroid nebulizer treatments daily. His parents were deathly afraid of him getting sick again because he had to be hospitalized twice. His birth history and infancy were unremarkable. I asked when he got his first pneumonia. His first infection was at 2 years of age. I asked what trauma happened to him at 15 or 18 months of age. His mother's eyes widened; she informed me that he fell from his father's shoulder backward onto pavement at 18 months. She even heard a loud "crack." Six months later, he got his first pneumonia. This was not a coincidence.

Upon physical examination, the ribs attached at the upper back were tight and stuck up. This means that in each breath, his exhalation is limited. It also means that in each inhalation, the ribs are not free to move higher. His effective air flow is poor. I checked his head and the area of the third diaphragm was tight and jammed. On his first treatment, I worked to free up all three diaphragms. They returned the following week with his mother reporting that his daily wheezing had stopped. Now, she asked if I could stop the daily chronic cough. Two weeks later, she reported that the coughing had stopped. I showed her the movement of his rib cage. He might need another treatment later when he has a growth spurt, which we'll know if he starts coughing again.

ALLERGIES

Allergies can appear at any age and vary in their presentation from mild to severe, in several tissue areas. There is an inherited familial genetic tendency involved in allergies. In infants and children, it can start off with itchy dry skin (called eczema) and/or chronic nasal congestion. In childhood, allergies tend to manifest as sensitivities to foods. A good, safe, and cheap way of controlling these early symptoms of food allergies is food elimination. As children age, that allergic tendency can change from food to respiratory triggers. The conventional medical approach is to recommend lifestyle changes and present a pharmaceutical solution. If the allergy episodes are few and far between, most people don't mind taking pills. But when the quality of one's life is affected by daily symptoms, the patient wants to learn more. When the conventional pharmaceutical approach becomes "prevention with steroids," many people start to ask about other options. Along with the usual dietary eliminations and environmental, home, and sleep changes that we recommend, traditional osteopathy can also offer a variety of options.

Mechanical restrictions can affect how our symptoms present. In infants and children the airway is so small that any amount of compression can cause issues with airflow and drainage. Over-reaction from an allergy response leads to mucus overproduction. Trauma or compression can lead to poor drainage and patients experience tissue congestion. Cranial osteopathic treatments usually help to open up the airway, allowing for drainage and flow.

In cases of severe allergic responses called anaphylaxis where tissue swelling risks airway compromise, most parents and patients feel helpless. They are given an epinephrine auto-injector (Epipen) to use in case of life-threatening allergic reactions. Currently, we do not have an answer for how or why sensitive patients overreact. Worse, we cannot predict which patients are likely to become these sensitive individuals.

Often, when I see cases of severe allergic reaction, I think that the white cells that patrol the body are extremely overreactive. They must have received their extreme marching orders from some tissue that is under stress. We know that white cells in the immune system are created in the marrow. They are sent out into the bloodstream to spend some time in certain tissue areas to be "primed," where they are educated, meaning that the cells are presented with a protein and programmed to recognize it as "foreign." Most of the time, this education occurs in lymphoid tissues such as the spleen, the adenoids, and lymph nodes. However, science has become increasingly aware of that some of these marching orders are being sent by the hypothalamus, an area deep in our brain, just behind our eyes and above our pituitary. So, when I see severe cases of allergy, I think of hypothalamic whiplash and blunt-force head trauma.

Theo is a 9-year-old boy who has always been allergic to peanuts. Every year he needs an update on his prescription for his Epipen. One year, his mother wanted to try traditional osteopathy to see if it could help. He had a history of difficult birth and head trauma, with a concussion several years prior. When I treated him his head felt very stuck and heavy. Several months later, his mother reported that the one visit really helped. She stated that in the past at the dinner table if she put down a plate sprinkled with just a little bit of peanuts, he would complain of nasal irritation. She actually thought he was faking. After the treatment, he could tolerate sitting nearby a dish with peanuts.

He had several more cranial osteopathic treatments whenever he exhibited negative behaviors or irritability. I told his mother to bring him in whenever he is especially "mean" to her, or evidences other types of abnormally negative or hostile behavior. He has had a total of six visits and they are happy with his progress. One day, they ate at a fast food restaurant where the food was cooked in peanut oil. His lips swelled mildly and responded readily to Benadryl®. He did not go into anaphylaxis and he did not use his Epipen. We all agreed, that even though he is better, he should always have the Epipen handy.

Another person whose unusual case of anaphylaxis I still marvel at is Lea. At 34 years of age, out of nowhere, she developed anaphylaxis and had to go to the ER. Every year for the last 3 years, she has needed an ER visit for steroid injections. During this same period, she starts developing boils. This is not a coincidence. Her immune system was going haywire. It is overreacting to a dangerous degree, while being lax in patrolling for foreign invaders. She came in to see if we could prevent the boils from cropping up. She feared that, within the next 4 months, she would have another reaction. We spent about eight visits trying to correct the boils, to no avail. Finally, on the last visit, we went over her trauma history again. No car accidents, no blunt force head trauma; I asked her again, because every little trauma counts. We went back to high school, junior high, and elementary school. Further back in childhood she recalls a bicycle accident. She was 2 years old, sitting on the front basket or handlebars of her dad's bicycle when they crashed. She has no memory of the event, but she recalls the family sitting around the table laughing over her maneuverings. She broke her leg in the accident and was casted. She could not walk well and so she went down the stairs on her buttocks at each step over the course of 6 weeks as a 2-year-old.

I reasoned that repetitive compressive loading from the sacrum up into the abdomen, as a result of this method of descending the stairs, was causing congestion in the spleen. The spleen is an organ tucked behind the stomach, on the upper left part of the abdomen. It is an organ where white blood cells also spend some time. I checked her spleen, and it felt tight and congested. Twenty minutes later, she felt and I sensed, simultaneously, a softening in the organ. I checked up with her a year later, and she no longer has allergic reactions or boils.

PART IV

HOW TO HELP OR FIND HELP FOR YOUR CHILD

PART IV: OVERVIEW

Each osteopathic treatment is an educational experience, for both patient and physician. Once a new patient experiences osteopathic manipulative treatment, they recognize that it is unlike the conventional philosophy of Western allopathic medicine, and is certainly quite different from any alternative physical therapy approach. With this newfound understanding of the lost art of traditional osteopathy, patients now have another option of healing from which to choose.

CHAPTER 15

Self-Care

To summarize this book, a mother now has more to stress and worry about than just feeding the baby and planning for college. Any trauma in the intervening years may very well derail or send the child on a tangential path through the medical system. Our job is to anticipate and prevent injury. Accidents do happen, we just have to have the knowledge and foresight to minimize risks and prevent them.

Planning and anticipating for minimizing risk starts off as early as planning to start a family. If the maternal pelvis has had trauma, that trauma should be treated and reduced prior to conception. If the treatment has been adequate, we should have resolution of symptoms of pain, gait should be unrestricted, and patients should have normal ovulatory cycles. Any musculoskeletal pains and medical problems not addressed and stabilized may make for a more difficult pregnancy and become destabilized during the second to last trimester, where weight and mechanical changes are most dramatic.

In pregnancy, the treated uterus should be able to expand to accommodate a single baby. The baby should be able to float and move around freely within the womb. By 35 weeks, the baby's head is growing rapidly and should be able to flip and position head down. If it cannot, should version, or turning the baby to point head-down, be attempted? If so, how many times? If the traumatized maternal pelvis is not adequately treated, the pregnancy may be less than ideal. Should one consider planning a C-section to mitigate these risks? Often, for the traumatized maternal uterus having difficulty with a pregnancy, the therapy is birth. A C-section is a highly controlled birth, the goal of which is to minimize injury to the mother and infant.

CHAPTER 16

Infancy

ONCE THE baby is home, the risks in the environment should be minimized. In the first years, falls and rolls off a short distance can influence development. So it makes sense to reduce these risks. Some general rules to live by:

1. No changing tables. Always change baby on the floor. I recommend purchasing a changing table pad and placing it on the floor.

2. Never turn your back on your baby. Always be mindful about falls and rolls and always keep your hands in contact with your baby.

3. Most of the rambunctious, active, climbing children (mostly boys, but occasionally girls) will have to be watched constantly.

4. Support of the infant's head and neck should always be with the hands. Often I see parents carry their baby with the head on the "crook of the elbow." And then the baby is rocked. This area in the back of the head and neck is delicate. The adult bony arm can end up cramming this delicate area and molding it tight. The supporting hand should be wide open with fingers splayed out. The thumb and index finger should support the head while the palm spans the delicate neck area. The ring and pinky fingers should be down at the level of the infant's shoulder blades.

5. When nursing, use a pillow to support the baby. Then use your arms to sweep the pillow with the baby up toward you to nurse. This will be less work and stress for both mother and infant.

If the baby has problems such as latching and nursing issues, fussiness, failure to thrive, what is to be done?
My first legal responsibility is to tell you to take your child to a pediatrician. If you are not happy with that pediatrician, find another. Then if you are not satisfied and do not get the results you seek, my second recommendation is for you to find an osteopathic physician near you. If the nearest osteopathic physician is far away, call and ask for a phone consultation. Some may charge and some may not. After your discussion, you will then have to decide if a drive is worth it. Get recommendations from parents in your support groups, church groups, or social network.

Once an accident or injury occurs, what can be done?
The safest thing to do after a medical evaluation for a fall or injury is to do nothing; just observe. If it was a minor injury, you and your child will forget about it. More spills and more minor injuries will eventually add up. At some point in time, sleep or behavior will be affected. Most of the time, this occurs with growth spurts. You can observe and time it exactly. Their appetites increase, they eat more, and they will need new clothes and shoes. Their feet, legs, and hamstrings will be tight. They have problems and can't stretch well. They won't tell you because they don't know and are not aware enough to tell you. You can do a physical inspection and once you observe the arched lower back, the high arches, or flattened out arches, you can check the tightness of the hamstrings or deep pelvic muscles. Once medical or behavioral issues arise, recall past traumas and seek out care. Then make an informed choice for how you want the care to be delivered and by whom.

What about furniture? How should I baby-proof my home?
Accidents happen. When it comes to the safety of children, I always advise minimizing risks by minimizing the chances of injury. As

previously stated, I have seen children fall off changing tables, and indeed it makes good sense to not even own a changing table. Believe it or not, the sleep arrangements should be focused on being as low to the ground as possible. One mattress placed directly on the floor is not only sufficient, it's also the safest. Bunk beds are great space savers, but they are also dangerous; I have seen too many injuries result from bunk beds, injuries that are truly life altering.

CHAPTER 17

Exercise for the Child

P HYSICAL ACTIVITY and cardiovascular exercise is important
for the human body. After an injury, there should be a period of
rest, then a return to activity, re-introduced slowly depending on
the severity of the injury.

In the older child, exercise habits of stretching and warming up and
warming down are a good routine to develop and keep consistent. As
with adults and seniors, being active and staying active is important in
overall health.

In the younger child, as the body is attempting to stretch out, there
are several activities parents can do with their children to improve range
of motion. One of the safest things I show parents to do is bicycling the
legs. For an infant, bicycling gets the legs moving. The babies love the
physical motion, and they enjoy the interaction. It is good fun and good
bonding time.

At any age, bicycling the legs is a good test of range of motion of
the legs and hips. When someone else moves the legs, the movements
should be smooth. Parents can usually feel tightness in the legs. When
range of motion catches repeatedly in one direction, try testing the
movement in another direction. If it is easier, continue along that
path. I instruct parents to follow what their child's body wants, then
after that, take the motion in the opposite direction. Most parents are

amazed to realize how much easier it is to allow the child to do what he or she wants; then and only then will the child's body allow a little more freedom in the opposite direction than it had previously. When following the patient, your child's path of least resistance is what we osteopaths call the "Direction of Ease." Many osteopathic physicians name their practice style, their practice, and their business using this term. It sounds so gentle and innocuous but it belies a powerful secret of traditional osteopathy. The body will only allow what it wants. There is no other way. For an effective treatment and for a therapeutic event to occur, we have to listen to what the body wants first and to then engage it, before it allows disengagement.

For children 5 years of age and older, I also instruct parents on the use of a neck exercise called a specific vector reduction (VRE); see below. I use it specifically for children who have had procedural interventions like intubation and dental procedures, and I do not generally apply it as regular form of exercise. The neck is a very specialized, still undeveloped area in children under ten. I very rarely treat or even touch this area in infants and children, because there are too many unformed neck bones forming from too many different pieces. I always advise against massage in this area for infants and children (and in adults as well, for that matter).

SPORTS

Exercise is not the same as sports. Getting out and playing are what children do best. Most kids know how to run around. Left to their own devices, most kids will do fine at a public park. Most parents will not agree with my recommending against any organized form of sports or league as a form of exercise. As they grow up, if the child and parent agree on a sport, the risks of injury and trauma are generally known and already accepted. It is not my purpose to dissuade, disagree, or make a judgement. My role is to educate both parents and patients regarding the repetitive stress on the body and to be available to provide osteopathic treatment of injuries. Parents need to know that traumas at the earliest stages of development can affect the child's development and alter it.

SPECIFIC VECTOR REDUCTION EXERCISES FOR ADULTS

The strain patterns of dental procedures (which are identical to the strain patterns of intubation) can benefit from certain routine exercises. I send all of my adult patients home with instructions for specific Vector Reduction Exercises (VREs), as well as a recommended sleep positioning advice. These exercises can easily correct a child's strain, even in children as young as 5 years old. Most types of head and neck injuries in life also mimic the strains of the dental chair and intubation, in that they cause the head and neck to be hyperextended. Patients who have whiplashed their neck will also respond well to these exercises. Note that it is always a good idea to perform a pre-exercise test of taking a deep breath, then inhaling through the nose.

Neck: Keeping an awareness of the back molars, gently bite the back teeth together and tuck your chin down. While doing both, add in a turning of the head from side to side. If it is more difficult to turn to one side than the other, always start with the easier side first.

Shoulders: Roll your shoulders back two times, and then roll them forward. Always start with a backward roll before the forward roll. Once both shoulders have been stretched this way, add the neck exercise component while continuing to do the shoulders. Try to do everything all at once.

Legs: As with children, adults can also benefit from bicycling of the legs. This helps free up the deep pelvic muscles that affect walking. Patients can use this exercise as a range of motion test to see if they have an old childhood rolling injury.

Hips: Lay down. Plant the feet flat so that the knees are bent up. Gently and slowly allow the thighs to fall to one side. Compare the range of motion; if one is tighter than the other, some injury at one time occurred. Always start with the side that is the easiest to do. Most of us have a tendency to roll off to our right; a good test would thus be to let the knees fall over to the right. If the left low back or hip lifts up off the bed or floor, then that side is tight. Stop if there is any tension whatsoever, and stop before there is any pain. Repeat for the left. If the right hip and low back lift up, this implies that the muscles are tight and on tension *as a unit*. Repeat multiple times.

You will see that any side that is tight will be just a little freer. With repetition (within the range that is allowed by the tight tissues), there should be a little more freedom each time as the range *increases*. Once the range of motion increases, the deep pelvic tension will let go, the gait will be easier, and the legs will feel lighter. Depending on the age, degree of injury, and types of injuries, this may only need to be done several times a day, though it may also be necessary for weeks, even months; perhaps for the rest of one's lifetime. Once the muscles are freed up (with the knees up while the feet stay planted), the next challenge is to bring the knee to one's chest. While holding on to the knees with the hands so that minimal work is required from the legs, testing from side to side will reveal more deep pelvic and low back tensions. Repeat.

Some patients are so tight that as soon as they pull their legs up, the lower ribs start to buck up. Worse still is when the chin and nose buck up into the air. This is evidence of a very tight backside, all the way from head to toe. Most patients cannot tell that they do this; they have no awareness of the tightness. The bucking up ribs, chin, and nose reflects an automatic, subconscious attempt to reduce tensions. I suggest that on one's first attempt you should have another person observe this automatic response. If this happens, it means that the knees are pulled too high up. Lower them a bit *without* using muscular effort in the legs; use of the arms and hands to lower the legs is preferable. Repeat. The final challenge is to engage the neck and hip exercises together, at the same time.

CHAPTER 18

Sleep Positioning

T HE IDEAL sleep position for the human body is lying on one's back, in what is medically termed "anatomic." This is when we lie on our backs with our legs shoulder width apart and our palms up. Most injured patients cannot do this. Some who can start out in this position may shift in the middle of the night and find themselves on their sides. If the above exercises are done correctly, the patient should be able to keep this sleep position longer through the night.

PILLOW POSITIONING

As previously mentioned, it is my absolute firm belief that pillows are to be used to support the head, and *not* the neck and shoulders. I believe most of us are doing it wrong; that what most of us do is intended to subconsciously splint old hyperextension neck injuries, whether they were acquired slowly and repetitively, or acutely. The ideal state and relationship of our heads on our necks while lying on a soft bed is one in which our necks are flexible and pliable enough to be flat without need of support. Medical conditions that require propping up of the head and neck include reflux, sinus congestion, and allergies, with or without a postnasal drip. From my osteopathic philosophical perspective, no medical condition is an exception to my rule. Rather, the question that should be asked is, "What mechanical cause is responsible for these conditions at all?" Once the medical conditions remit or improve, then the pillow issue may more readily be addressed.

If a pillow is necessary, what would be the proper position? The lower edge of the pillow should touch the area of the head behind the ears. When sleeping on one's back, there should be a space in between the area just above the neck, all the way down to the shoulders. This space allows for the neck to stretch throughout the night.

There is one final step in the treatment of head and neck hyperextension. After doing the above exercises for the neck and hips, just before drifting off to sleep, I instruct patients to bite the back molars, tuck the chin and push the back of the head into the *properly placed* pillow. This last step will initiate sleep and allow stretching of the neck muscles overnight.

FETAL SLEEP POSITIONING OR FETAL SLEEPING FOR THE ADULT

In our early development, if womb conditions are ideal, peaceful, and protective, the fetus has its head down and chin tucked. In this position, the back of the neck is stretched and its resting length is much longer (relative to our size) than at any other time in our skeletally mature adult lives. I have come to the conclusion that this position is even more effective than sleeping with the head and neck flat on the bed. For 9 months and 2 weeks (under ideal scenarios), we are in this position. It is our earliest position, after we are transformed from a flat sheet to a tube that rounds out at the top of the head and at the bottom at our tailbone. In living out our adult lives and in surviving our injuries, we are always moving away from this position. We no longer consciously remember this fetal sleep position.

If you were successful in reducing hyperextension in your head and neck using the above Vector Reduction Exercises, there is one final test. Fetal sleeping is the final summit in attaining neck freedom. Napping in an upright position tends to be difficult. Most of us reflexively reach for a pillow for head and neck support. Once in place, we tend to sleep with our head and neck hyperextended. Instead of putting it back and up, your head should be hanging forward, providing for a more restful nap than one might expect. Upon waking, you may experience some stiffness around your forehead and temple area, but this should soon release. The feeling this creates in the back of the neck is one of profound freedom, with no tension whatsoever.

Some words of caution: only adults who have succeeded with the prior exercises should attempt fetal sleeping. Jumping straight into fetal sleeping may be too abrupt, and some people may experience side effects. Fetal sleeping should not be attempted with children, as they are still skeletally immature, and their airway is smaller and shorter.

CHAPTER 19

Finding an Osteopath

W HEN I search for a colleague to refer friends and family of my patients to, I guide them as to how to continue that search and narrow it down. The general rule I apply is that they should find someone who has been in practice for a long time. After seven or so years in practice, the skills and philosophical concepts are so automatic and ingrained that whatever questions you have, your osteopathic physician should be able to answer in a way that gives you a sense of confidence. Generally for most of us, we get better with age and experience. Our professional skill increases with age, like a fine wine. The second question to ask is whether they practice traditional osteopathy some, or most, of the time. The more experienced of us tend to do a lot of traditional osteopathy a lot of the time. One cannot just *like* osteopathy. Those who do this for a living *love* it; we respect it profoundly and wholeheartedly. The best way to choose your doctor is to call and talk or ask for a consultation. Most of us do not take insurance. It is always best to do your research and ask questions.

WHAT TO EXPECT

In general, we usually advise that whatever course of treatment you choose, do one at a time so that you can see the effect. Whatever happens to the physical body, the organism, the patient will adapt as best it can. Support at any stage is helpful, if treatment is not available. With the exception of plagiocephaly and torticollis, watchful waiting is a reasonable conservative approach. If you find a traditional osteopathic physician, precision work should show results within the week, if not the same day.

I usually request that patients complete whatever other forms of structural therapy they are currently doing before coming to see me. It would not make sense to have multiple hands-on treatment and mixing regimens, traveling between osteopathic physician, chiropractor, and physical therapist.

FINAL THOUGHTS

OPEFULLY, BY this time, you have gained an understanding that structural imbalances can cause multiple medical issues that by conventional standards would be considered unrelated. Throughout this book, I hope I have successfully tied multiple issues of seemingly complex cases down to a few causative structural strains.

When you find the right doctor for you or your child you will know because unexpected changes will happen. Things that you had not thought to mention or had completely forgotten will be addressed. It may also be that the issue seems minor compared to the current medical problem and too frequently may seem too bothersome to mention—much like Rachel, who came to me for migraines while also suffering from a painful indented right shin. To this day, she is still very happy and remembers the one visit where she was cured of that shin pain.

Through my own journey to understanding my structural issues, I too remember an unexpected cure. To this day I remain grateful to my colleague, Robert Trafeli, D.O. We were addressing the old issues of my left eye and he found an old issue of the fourth toe of my left foot. I had so many other things going on, that was the last item I would ever hope to clear up. For about 15 years that toe, in certain positions, would without warning go into a painful debilitating spasm. He found it, and he fixed it. I no longer have to live in fear of positioning the foot incorrectly lest it seize up. All these years, I lived under the impression that my whole right side was severely altered from my minor car accident. I now believe the left side was just as bad or maybe even worse. That persistently troubling toe was a hint that the true cause of most of my problems came from above, to the left. That one little accident, from 27 years ago, did so much more than I ever realized (yes, high velocity injuries will have that kind of a long lasting semi-permanence to them).

When you find the right doctor for you or your child, my hope is that you gain more understanding of how our structural body shapes us, not just physically but also emotionally. Will that translate into peace of mind and happiness with who we are? Will we be more patient and forgiving of ourselves and of others? Once we understand that the person we come to be is shaped by all that has happened to our physical bodies and the challenges it presents, can we come to an appreciation of the beauty in this life?

Good luck to you on your journey in finding the cause of who you are, in understanding and minimizing trauma risks for your children, and in seeking help and getting answers.

RESOURCES

AMERICAN OSTEOPATHIC ASSOCIATION

Chicago Office (Main Headquarters)
142 E. Ontario St.
Chicago, IL 60611-2864
Toll-free phone: (800) 621-1773
General phone: (312) 202-8000
Fax: (312) 202-8200

Washington, D.C. Office
1090 Vermont Ave. NW, Ste. 500
Washington, D.C. 20005
Toll-free phone: (800) 962-9008
General phone: (202) 414-0140
Fax: (202) 544-3525

CRANIAL ACADEMY

3535 E. 96th Street, Suite 101
Indianapolis, IN 46240
Office Phone: 317-581-0411
Office Fax: 317-580-9299
E-mail: info@cranialacademy.org

AMERICAN ACADEMY OF OPTOMETRY

2909 Fairgreen Street
Orlando, Florida 32803
Phone: (321) 710-EYES (3937)
Toll-Free: (800) 969-4226
Fax: (407) 893-9890
Email: aaoptom@aaoptom.org
Website: http://www.aaopt.org

AMERICAN OPTOMETRIC FOUNDATION (OF)

2909 Fairgreen Street
Orlando, Florida 32803
Phone: (321) 710-3937
Toll-Free: (800) 368-6263
Fax: (407) 893-9890
Email: aof@aaoptom.org

COLLEGE OF OPTOMETRISTS
IN VISION DEVELOPMENT

215 W. Garfield Rd, Ste 200
Aurora, OH 44202
Phone: (330) 995-0718
Fax: (330) 995-0719
www.covd.org
Email: info@covd.org

NEURO-OPTOMETRIC REHABILITATION ASSOCIATION

28514 Constellation Road
Valencia, CA 91355
Phone: (949) 250-0176
Email: info@nora.cc

For vision therapy in Los Angeles:

HOLLYWOOD VISION CENTER

Optometrist Brisco Elise, OD
955 Carrillo Dr Ste 105, Los Angeles, CA 90048
Phone: (323) 954-5800

For vision therapy in the San Gabriel Valley:

CENTER FOR VISION DEVELOPMENT OPTOMETRY

Derek Tong, O.D., FAAO, FCOVD, FNORA
2700 E. Foothill Blvd., Ste. 207, Pasadena, CA 91107
Phone: (626) 578-9685

REFERENCES

1 http://www.bls.gov/oes/current/oes291123.htm#(1).

2 Chapman-Smith, David. *The Chiropractic Profession: Its Education, Practice, Research and Future Directions*. West Des Moines, Iowa: NCMIC Group, Inc. p. 25.

3 Homola S. "Chiropractic: History and overview of theories and methods." *Clin Orthop Relat Res*. 2006 Mar;444:236–42.

4 Chapman-Smith, David. *The Chiropractic Profession: Its Education, Practice, Research and Future Directions*. West Des Moines, Iowa: NCMIC Group, Inc. pp 67-70.

5 https://www.acatoday.org/content_css.cfm?CID=3077 (chiropractic acupuncture).

6 http://www.upledger.com/content.asp?id=26.

7 https://nmtcenter.com/history/#euro.

8 http://www.bls.gov/ooh/healthcare/massage-therapists.htm.

9 Mainous RO, "Infant massage as a component of developmental care: past, present, and future." *Holist Nurs Pract*. 2002 Oct;16(5):1–7.

10 Field T, "Massage therapy." *Med Clin North Am*. 2002 Jan;86(1):163–1.

11 www.drdeanhowell.com.

12 http://www.cdc.gov/traumaticbraininjury/get_the_facts.html.

13 http://www-nrd.nhtsa.dot.gov/Pubs/812101.pdf.

14 LaGasse LL1, Neal AR, Lester BM. "Assessment of infant cry: acoustic cry analysis and parental perception." *Ment Retard Dev Disabil Res Rev.* 2005;11(1):83–93.

15 Sisto R, Bellieni CV, Perrone S, Buonocore G. "Neonatal pain analyzer: development and validation." *Med Biol Eng Comput.* 2006 Oct;44(10):841–5. Epub 2006 Sep 16.

16 Vaz I. "Probable trigeminal autonomic cephalgia in a 3-month-old male infant." *Dev Med Child Neurol.* 2010 Apr;52(4):400–2. doi: 10.1111/j.1469-8749.2009.03532.x. Epub 2009 Dec 9.

17 Gelfand AA, Goadsby PJ, Allen IE. *Cephalalgia.* 2015 Jan;35(1):63–72. doi: 10.1177/0333102414534326. Epub 2014 May 22. "The relationship between migraine and infant colic: a systematic review and meta-analysis."

18 Landgren K, Lundqvist A, Hallström I. *Open Nurs J.* 2012;6:53–61. doi: 10.2174/1874434601206010053. Epub 2012 May 2. "Remembering the Chaos — But Life Went on and the Wound Healed. A Four-Year Follow-Up with Parents having had a Baby with Infantile Colic."

19 Yoganandan N1, Pintar FA, Lew SM, Rao RD, Rangarajan N. "Quantitative analyses of pediatric cervical spine ossification patterns using computed tomography." *Ann Adv Automot Med.* 2011;55:159–68.

20 http://www.stanfordchildrens.org/en/topic/default?id=sports-injury-statistics-90-P02787.

21 Pinyerd BJ. "Strategies for consoling the infant with colic: Fact or fiction?" *J Pediatr Nurs.* 1992 Dec;7(6):403–11.

22 Gelfand AA, Thomas KC, Goadsby PJ. "Before the headache: Infant colic as an early life expression of migraine." *Neurology.* 2012 Sep 25;79(13):1392–6. Epub 2012 Sep 12.

23 Romanello S1, Spiri D, Marcuzzi E, Zanin A, Boizeau P, Riviere S, Vizeneux A, Moretti R, Carbajal R, Mercier JC, Wood C, Zuccotti GV, Crichiutti G, Alberti C, Titomanlio L. "Association between childhood migraine and history of infantile colic." *JAMA*. 2013 Apr 17;309(15):1607–12. doi: 10.1001/jama.2013.747.

24 Sillanpää M, Saarinen M. "Infantile colic associated with childhood migraine: A prospective cohort study." *Cephalalgia*. 2015 Mar 9. pii: 0333102415576225. [Epub ahead of print]

25 Kim JS. *Korean J Pediatr*. 2011 Jun;54(6):229–33. doi: 10.3345/kjp.2011.54.6.229. Epub 2011 Jun 30. "Excessive crying: behavioral and emotional regulation disorder in infancy."

26 Schwartz CE, Kunwar PS, Greve DN, Moran LR, Viner JC, Covino JM, Kagan J, Stewart SE, Snidman NC, Vangel MG, Wallace SR. *Arch Gen Psychiatry*. 2010 Jan;67(1):78–84. doi: 10.1001/archgen-psychiatry.2009.171. "Structural differences in adult orbital and ventromedial prefrontal cortex predicted by infant temperament at 4 months of age."

27 Lobo ML, Kotzer AM, Keefe MR, Brady E, Deloian B, Froese-Fretz A, Barbosa G. J "Current beliefs and management strategies for treating infant colic." *Pediatr Health Care*. 2004 May–Jun;18(3):115–22.

28 Douglas PS, Hill PS. *Curr Opin Pediatr*. 2011 Oct;23(5):523–9. doi: 10.1097/MOP.0b013e32834a1b78. "The crying baby: what approach?"

29 Hiscock, H. Aust Fam Physician. 2006 Sep;35(9):680–4. "The crying baby."

30 Hewson P, Oberklaid F, Menahem S. "Infant colic, distress, and crying." *Clin Pediatr* (Phila). 1987 Feb;26(2):69–76.

31 Owens ME. "Pain in infancy: conceptual and methodological issues." *Pain*. 1984 Nov;20(3):213–30.

32 Rimer R, Hiscock H. *J Paediatr Child Health.* 2014 Mar;50(3):202–7. doi: 10.1111/jpc.12452. Epub 2013 Dec 23. "National survey of Australian paediatricians' approach to infant crying."

33 Biggs WS. "Diagnosis and management of positional head deformity." *Am Fam Physician.* 2003 May 1;67(9):1953–6.

34 Kane AA, Mitchell LE, Craven KP, Marsh JL. "Observations on a recent increase in plagiocephaly without synostosis." *Pediatrics.* 1996 Jun;97(6 Pt 1):877–85.

35 Turk AE, McCarthy JG, Thorne CH, Wisoff JH. "The 'back to sleep campaign' and deformational plagiocephaly: Is there cause for concern?" *J Craniofac Surg.* 1996 Jan;7(1):12–8.

36 Wilbrand JF, Wilbrand M, Malik CY, Howaldt HP, Streckbein P, Schaaf H, Kerkmann H. "Complications in helmet therapy." *J Craniomaxillofac Surg.* 2012 Jun;40(4):341–6. doi: 10.1016/j.jcms.2011.05.007. Epub 2011 Jul 8.

37 Roby BB1, Finkelstein M, Tibesar RJ, Sidman JD. "Prevalence of positional plagiocephaly in teens born after the 'Back to Sleep' campaign." *Otolaryngol Head Neck Surg.* 2012 May;146(5):823–8. doi: 10.1177/0194599811434261. Epub 2012 Jan 12.

38 Collett BR, Gray KE, Starr JR, Heike CL, Cunningham ML, Speltz ML. "Development at age 36 months in children with deformational plagiocephaly." *Pediatrics.* 2013 Jan;131(1):e109–15. doi: 10.1542/peds.2012-1779. Epub 2012 Dec 24.

39 Collett BR, Starr JR, Kartin D, Heike CL, Berg J, Cunningham ML, Speltz ML. "Development in toddlers with and without deformational plagiocephaly." *Arch Pediatr Adolesc Med.* 2011 Jul;165(7):653–8. doi: 10.1001/archpediatrics.2011.92.

40 Shamji MF, Fric-Shamji EC, Merchant P, Vassilyadi M. "Cosmetic and cognitive outcomes of positional plagiocephaly treatment." *Clin Invest Med.* 2012 Oct 6;35(5):E266.

41 Kordestani RK, Patel S, Bard DE, Gurwitch R, Panchal J. "Neurodevelopmental delays in children with deformational plagiocephaly." *Plast Reconstr Surg.* 2006 Jan;117(1):207–18; discussion 219–20.

42 Hutchison BL1, Stewart AW, de Chalain T, Mitchell EA. "Serial developmental assessments in infants with deformational plagiocephaly." *J Paediatr Child Health.* 2012 Mar;48(3):274–8. doi: 10.1111/j.1440-1754.2011.02234.x. Epub 2011 Nov 14.

43 Stellwagen L1, Hubbard E, Chambers C, Jones KL. "Torticollis, facial asymmetry and plagiocephaly in normal newborns." *Arch Dis Child.* 2008 Oct;93(10):827–31. doi: 10.1136/adc.2007.124123. Epub 2008 Apr 1.

44 Sergueef N, Nelson KE, Glonek T. "Palpatory diagnosis of plagiocephaly." *Complement Ther Clin Pract.* 2006 May;12(2):101–10. Epub 2006 Mar 29.

45 Lessard S1, Gagnon I, Trottier N. "Exploring the impact of osteopathic treatment on cranial asymmetries associated with nonsynostotic plagiocephaly in infants." *Complement Ther Clin Pract.* 2011 Nov;17(4):193–8. doi: 10.1016/j.ctcp.2011.02.001. Epub 2011 Mar 5.

46 Cerritelli F, Martelli M, Renzetti C, Pizzolorusso G, Cozzolino V, Barlafante G. "Introducing an osteopathic approach into neonatology ward: the NE-O model." *Chiropr Man Therap.* 2014 May 9;22:18. doi: 10.1186/2045-709X-22-18. eCollection 2014.

47 http://www.drweil.com/drw/u/ART00348/ear-infections.html.

48 Spiegal DA, Dormans JP *Kliegman: Nelson Textbook of Pediatrics,* 19th ed., 2011 Philadelphia, PA: Elsevier

49 Johan Emil Lange, Harald Steen, Ragnhild Gunderson, and Jens Ivar Brox "Long-term results after Boston brace treatment in late-onset juvenile and adolescent idiopathic scoliosis." *Scoliosis.* 2011; 6: 18. Published online 2011 August 31. doi: 10.1186/1748-7161-6-18.

50 Renshaw TS. "The role of Harrington instrumentation and posterior spine fusion in the management of adolescent idiopathic scoliosis." *Orthop Clin North Am.* 1988 Apr;19(2):257–67.

51 Radice-Neumann D, Zupan B, Babbage DR, Willer B. "Overview of impaired facial affect recognition in persons with traumatic brain injury." *Brain Inj.* 2007 Jul;21(8):807–16.

52 Barlow K, Thompson E, Johnson D, Minns RA. "The neurological outcome of non-accidental head injury." *Pediatr Rehabil.* 2004 Jul-Sep;7(3):195–203.

53 Gregory SG, Anthopolos R, Osgood CE, Grotegut CA, Miranda ML. "Association of autism with induced or augmented childbirth in North Carolina Birth Record (1990–1998) and Education Research (1997–2007) databases." *JAMA Pediatr.* 2013 Oct;167(10):959–66. doi: 10.1001/jamapediatrics.2013.2904.

54 Yang WH, Jing J, Xiu LJ, Cheng MH, Wang X, Bao P, Wang QX. Regional cerebral blood flow in children with autism spectrum disorders: a quantitative 99mTc-ECD brain SPECT study with statistical parametric mapping evaluation." *Chin Med J* (Engl). 2011 May;124(9):1362–6.

55 Goldman S, O'Brien LM, Filipek PA, Rapin I, Herbert MR. "Motor stereotypies and volumetric brain alterations in children with Autistic Disorder." *Res Autism Spectr Disord.* 2013 Jan 1;7(1):82–92.

56 Blaylock RL. "Immunology primer for neurosurgeons and neurologists part 2: Innate brain immunity." *Surg Neurol Int.* 2013 Sep 18;4:118. doi: 10.4103/2152-7806.118349.

57 Herbert MR, Ziegler DA, Makris N, Filipek PA, Kemper TL, Normandin JJ, Sanders HA, Kennedy DN, Caviness VS Jr. "Localization of white matter volume increase in autism and developmental language disorder." *Ann Neurol.* 2004 Apr;55(4):530–40.

58 Granpeesheh D1, Tarbox J, Dixon DR, Carr E, Herbert M. "Retrospective analysis of clinical records in 38 cases of recovery from autism." *Ann Clin Psychiatry.* 2009 Oct–Dec;21(4):195–204.

59 Helt M, Kelley E, Kinsbourne M, Pandey J, Boorstein H, Herbert M, Fein D. "Can children with autism recover? If so, how?" *Neuropsychol Rev.* 2008 Dec;18(4):339–66. doi: 10.1007/s11065-008-9075-9. Epub 2008 Nov 14.

ABOUT THE AUTHOR

Dr. LeTrinh Hoang is a pediatrician in private practice offering holistic, integrative pediatrics. She has two offices where she combines homeopathy and osteopathy consultations. She is a graduate of the University of New England, College of Osteopathic Medicine (1997). She received her pediatrics training at Loma Linda University Children's Hospital (2000). Shortly thereafter, she returned to the study of traditional osteopathy, as it was intended by the founder of the profession, using a hands-on approach to diagnosing and treating the body.